<u>Cancer</u>
Balancing Reality and Hope

For the Newly Diagnosed & Those Who Love Them

by Alan Spector

Alan Spector

Copyright © by Alan Spector 2019

Contact the author for special quantity discounts

Alan Spector

BBallNever2Old@aol.com

ISBN: 978-1-79764-420-2

Also by Alan Spector

Baseball: Never Too Old to Play "The" Game

Hail Hail to U City High

Your Retirement Quest
(with coauthor Keith Lawrence)

University City Schools: Our First 100 Years

Body Not Recovered

After the Cheering Stops

www.aaspector.com

Alan Spector

Dedication

To the breadth and depth of the Cancer Community—to survivors and their loved ones, to dedicated medical professionals, researchers, advocates, and administrators, to supportive individuals and organizations, and to tireless fundraising organizations and their donors.

Specifically—to Doctors William Birenbaum, Gary Ratkin, and Nancy Bartlett and their staffs—I am here and writing this book because of you and for you.

And mostly—to my mother, Jeanette Friedman Spector, and my father, Herman Spector, both lost to cancer and both who lived full and meaningful lives.

Acknowledgments

Thank you, first and foremost, to my wife, Ann, my cancer support leader, forever cheerleader, and the willing wielder of your red editing pen.

Thank you to Louis DeGennaro, PhD, President and CEO of the Leukemia & Lymphoma Society, for your insights in the book's Foreword.

Thank you to the medical professionals who gave their time and insights to the development of the book: Dr. Nancy Bartlett, Dr. Rick Boulay, Dr. Nicole Giamanco, Dr. John Marshall, Laura Melton, PhD, Dr. Carissa Wood, and Susan Young, RN.

Thank you to the researchers and other professionals who also provided their time and insights: Cathy Bradley, PhD, Jan Bresch, Amy Burd, PhD, Betsy Clark, PhD, Mark Kochevar, MBA, Judy Mange, MBA/PT/CMC, Rajiv Mehta, Renata Sledge, MSW/LCSW, Rabbi Jeffrey Stiffman, Sister Carla Mae Streeter, O.P.

Thank you to relatives and friends old and new, who are survivors, loved ones, and cancer supporters for your encouragement, sensitivity, insights, and personal stories: Ronnie and Allen Brockman, Jill Chapin, Ron Doornink, Marti and Harvey Ferdman, Teri Griege, Rick Hitt, Bob Miller, Don Pearline, Bob Radinsky, Kevin Spector, and Carol Strelic.

A special thank you to those who were also beta-readers of the manuscript: Dr. Nancy Bartlett, Jill Chapin, Betsy Clark PhD, Marti Ferdman RN, Bob Radinsky, and Susan Young RN.

Alan Spector

Table of Contents

Foreword

When Alan asked me to write the Foreword for his book, I was delighted, because *Cancer: Balancing Reality and Hope* addresses a critical element of our mission at the Leukemia & Lymphoma Society, improving the lives of patients and their families.

The reality is that there is never a good time to get cancer, but the hope is that now, today, is a phenomenal time to be fighting it. There is increasing optimism that we are on the cusp of curing cancer, what has been called "the emperor of all maladies."

At LLS, we come face-to-face with blood cancer every day, and there are many other organizations similarly dedicated to fighting cancers of all types. We fund cutting-edge research, advocate for state and federal policies that benefit patients and their loved ones, and provide free information, support services, and financial assistance to those in need. We have invested more than $1.2 billion in blood-cancer research since being founded in 1949, and we provide information to and support for over 30,000 people each year.

Yet, despite our deep connection with all aspects of the disease, we are not nearly as close to it as are cancer patients and their loved ones. Whether diagnosed with blood cancer or one of the many other forms of the disease, they are the true fighters—those who are affected daily by the cancer itself, by the effects of the treatment regimens, by what some refer to as the "financial toxicity" of battling cancer, and by the emotional challenges that invariably accompany the experience.

At a time when it is most difficult to do so, each newly-diagnosed patient and each loved one has so many things to think about and so many decisions to make. Even if they have previously experienced cancer through a family member, friend, or colleague, a personal diagnosis is new and much more intense. With all the complexity they are and will be facing, it is not surprising that they are asking themselves and others, "Where can I learn what I need to know?"

In a world full of information, some good and some not so good, answering that question well is a major attraction of Alan's book. The title very well could have been, *Cancer: How to Think About What to Think About*. Although this book will be meaningful for any cancer patient and his or her caregiving loved ones, it is especially helpful for, as the subtitle states, *For the Newly Diagnosed & Those Who Love Them*.

Alan, himself a blood cancer survivor, has constructed a framework each patient and loved one can use to address their disease, regardless of their diagnosis and prognosis. That framework begins with acknowledging and addressing the reality of the disease—then it helps appreciate the value of building hope and provides an approach for doing so.

Importantly, Alan then brings it all together when he urges each cancer patient and each loved one to develop two personalized plans, their cancer plan and their non-cancer life plan. And he guides the reader through that process. This is but one of the unique features I found in the book. It builds from Alan's retirement life-planning expertise—he is the author of two books on the subject and conducts workshops around the country, helping people plan for the non-financial aspects of their retirements. In *Cancer: Balancing Reality and Hope*, Alan applies these life lessons to help each patient and loved one recognize that while cancer and the plan to address it can sometimes be all-consuming, there is also a non-cancer segment of life that can and should be enhanced.

It is Alan's first-person breadth of perspective that has enabled him to craft this book. As a nine-year blood cancer survivor and a strategic planning consultant, he has worked closely with the cancer research, medical, and support community for a decade; and for two decades he has studied, written about, and taught others about life planning.

Regardless of your diagnosis and prognosis, I urge you to delve into each section of the book: acknowledge your reality and address it; recognize the value of building hope and do so; and balance the two by creating and living both your cancer and non-cancer life plans.

Louis DeGennaro, Ph.D.
President and Chief Executive Officer
Leukemia & Lymphoma Society

Introduction

"I accept reality and dare not question it."
Walt Whitman

"Hope is being able to see that there is light despite all the darkness."
Desmond Tutu

"Have you had a cold?"

"No."

"Have you had an infection?"

"No, not that I know of. Why do you ask?"

"Your white blood count is slightly elevated. Let's make arrangements for you to see a hematologist just to make sure everything is OK."

This was an exchange between my primary care physician, Dr. William Birenbaum, and me during an annual physical.

Fast forward to the appointment with the hematologist. As I stride down the hallway, I'm focused on looking for his office, having no concerns—just another routine check. Why be concerned? Feel great. Physically fit—spending two hours in the gym four days a week. Age 64—still playing baseball; no, not softball; baseball. This is just another doctor's appointment "just to make sure everything is OK."

I find the office suite, enter, and am dumbstruck by one of the words above the receptionist's window, "ONCOLOGY." In the next hour, my blood is drawn, centrifuged, and analyzed. I am now sitting in Dr. Gary Ratkin's office, listening more-than-intently.

In a gentle caring tone, he explains, "White blood cells are created in the bone marrow and sent into the bloodstream to circulate around your body, poised to fight infection. If there is an infection, the body generates even more white cells. Inside each of these cells is a switch that eventually kills it off to make room for others. In some people, these switches stop working. We can tell from testing your blood, using flow cytometry, whether your high white count is a function of more cells being created to fight an infection or a function of the switches not working.

"In your case, the switches aren't working. Your white cells aren't dying off the way they are supposed to. In and of themselves, these extra white cells in your bloodstream and bone marrow are not an issue. However, if the counts increase sufficiently to be crowding out healthy white cells, red cells, and platelets, that can become a problem. If that happens, we would need to treat the condition. For now, the best thing to do is monitor your white count and other blood markers every three months to see how the numbers are progressing."

This is all making sense. It's logical. It's scientific. I get it. I've got this condition. We'll monitor it. If need be, we'll treat it. He's calm. I'm calm.

Then, before asking if I have any questions, he says, "There is a name for this condition. It's Chronic Lymphocytic Leukemia, sometimes referred to as CLL."

Wait! What? Leukemia? Isn't that blood cancer?

My logical engineering mind is now in conflict with my emotional what-do-you-mean-I-have-cancer mind, just as my white cells are now at war with the rest of my bloodstream. I've frequently heard the term "battling cancer." But now, it's about me. And already, I'm engaged in battles, none of them by choice.

When I get home from the doctor, my wife, Ann, reacts to the news with a comforting calm. Later she tells me that she was able to appear calm, because I had shared the details with her as Dr. Ratkin had explained them to me. By the time I got to the word "leukemia," she was convinced that I knew what we needed to do and felt that I believed everything would be OK. She also tells me that it went through her mind that if she weren't strong, I might feel as though I need to attend to her, when I should be fully focused on attending to myself.

Shortly thereafter, Dr. Ratkin retires and I begin seeing Dr. Nancy Bartlett at the Siteman Cancer Center in St. Louis, where I live. Three months after my first appointment with her and after a lot of reading about CLL, I return to Siteman, but I'm early for my scheduled blood draw and hands-on checkup to look for enlarged lymph nodes.

In the few minutes I have before heading toward the lab to have my blood drawn, I'm standing in front of the floor-to-ceiling Cancer Center windows overlooking the busy intersection of Forest Park Parkway and Euclid Avenue.

Among the pedestrians and drivers going to work, appointments, or wherever, there are about 100 people in my sun-lit morning view. Based on what I've learned from my reading, I realize that about 40 of those 100 people either already have been or will be diagnosed with some form of cancer during their lifetimes. And virtually every one of the 100 either knows or will know a relative or friend with the disease.

When experiencing the life-changing diagnosis, each of the intersection people and each of us, whether survivor or loved one, is confronted with three things simultaneously. There is the reality of the disease with all of its physical implications and its required decision-making. There is the inevitable rush of emotion. And there is the beginning of a relentless search for hope.

I just used the word "survivor" for the first time, so let's pause for a moment to establish the definition that we'll use interchangeably throughout the book with the word "patient." The term "survivor" has meant different things over the years, but currently, according to the National Cancer Institute of the National Institutes of Health, "a person is considered to be a survivor from the time of diagnosis until the end of life."

The definition is irrespective of the type of cancer, whether the cancer is acute or chronic, what its stage is, or what the prognosis is. It doesn't take into account how the person is tolerating or responding to treatment or emotionally coping with the disease. Basically, if you have been diagnosed, you are, by definition, a survivor.

That first discussion with Dr. Birenbaum took place in 2010. Until this book was published, only my immediate family, my medical support team, a couple of close friends, and a number of cancer researchers, knew about my CLL. But this book is not just about my coming out.

Rather it is about my mom, who died of ovarian cancer, and my dad, who died of lung cancer. It is about my mother-in-law, who is a 10+ year ovarian cancer survivor, and my brother-in-law, who is a 15+ year colorectal cancer survivor, with whom his doctor has used the word "cured." It is about the too-many relatives, classmates, friends, and others I know who have been diagnosed and are either survivors or not.

It is about my youngest sister, who is a dedicated and tireless nurse just like our mother, and my middle sister, who courageously and compassionately counsels others about grieving, death, and dying.

It is about all the spouses, partners, parents, children, and friends whose loved one has been diagnosed.

It is about all the dedicated people in the cancer research and care community, many of whom you'll meet throughout the book, as they have taken the time to share their insights.

It is about all of the countless volunteers and donors and fundraisers and advocates who give of their time, talent, and treasure to make a difference in our lives.

And it is about those 100 people outside the Siteman Cancer Center windows. Among them were likely cancer researchers, doctors, nurses, caregivers, and survivors. There was likely a father or mother or brother or sister or friend who had lost or would lose a loved one to the disease. And there were also likely many who were not yet affected—someone on his way to the corner coffee shop, a financial advisor on the way to her office, a construction worker going to the nearby site on which a hospital was being rebuilt.

But mostly it is about those living with cancer and those who love them, the spouse of someone newly diagnosed, the parents of a child survivor, a friend who learns of a diagnosis from 1000 miles away.

Although I felt compelled to write this book, before I began, I reflected on why I should do so and what value I might add to the many instructive cancer books already published. Said another way, what do I have to offer that would make this book worth your precious time to read and heed?

I concluded there were three reasons to proceed.

First—as a cancer survivor, I have a vested interest in the disease and more experience with it than I would choose to have. And I strive to be personally *Balancing Reality and Hope*.

Second—coincident with the timing of my personal cancer journey, I've had an opportunity to interact closely with what I referred to above as the broader cancer community in a different and more intimate way than most people. About the same time I was learning about my CLL, a former work colleague reached out to ask me if I was still involved with strategic planning, something he and I had done together at Procter & Gamble. As it turns out, since retiring, I had been doing strategic planning consulting for local nonprofits.

He was on the Board of the Prevent Cancer Foundation in Alexandria, Virginia, and they were interested in developing a strategic plan for their organization. Shortly thereafter, I was periodically traveling from St. Louis to help them meet their objectives. Through subsequent referrals, I have since consulted for the Ruesch Center for the Cure of Gastrointestinal Cancers and the Lombardi Comprehensive Cancer Center, both on the Georgetown University campus, the national Leukemia & Lymphoma Society in White Plains, New York, the University of Colorado Comprehensive Cancer Center, the Colorado Center for Personalized Medicine in Denver, and Fight Colorectal Cancer.

Through these engagements and my personal cancer experience, I have had the opportunity to meet and learn from dedicated researchers, medical professionals, funders, donors, administrators, advocates, caregivers, and others who individually and collectively make a difference in the lives of survivors and their loved ones.

Third—there is relevance to two of my previous six books, *Your Retirement Quest*, coauthored with my friend Keith Lawrence, who is the husband of a cancer survivor, and *After the Cheering Stops*. For more than a decade, through the books, workshops, and personal coaching, I have been helping individuals and couples develop meaningful plans for the critical nonfinancial aspects of their retirement lives. In the final chapters of this book, you'll have an opportunity to use those same life planning principles, concepts, and tools to develop your personalized plan for *Balancing Reality and Hope*.

Cancer is an equal-opportunity disease. A retired French engineer who has never smoked is diagnosed with lung cancer...a three-year old from Phoenix is diagnosed with leukemia...an African-American accountant, who is pregnant with her first child, is diagnosed with breast cancer, having lost a grandmother and aunt to the disease...a 50-year old Japanese computer engineer is diagnosed with multiple myeloma...a Midwestern oncology nurse in her 40s, having cared for thousands of cancer patients, is diagnosed with colorectal cancer...a vital 20-something major league baseball player is diagnosed with testicular cancer...

The loved ones of survivors are no less diverse—spouse, friend, daughter, brother, neighbor, colleague, parent, partner, pastor...

Each person, each cancer diagnosis, and each set of life circumstances are different. Yet, there are compelling common themes that run through each survivor's story. There is the reality of the diagnosis itself, of the effect it has on so many aspects of the life of the survivor and his or her loved ones, and of the emotions that ensue. There is the relentless quest for hope. And there is the value of *Balancing Reality and Hope* in a way that enables us to create and live our best lives.

The book is structured around those three themes, Reality, Hope, and Balance.

Reality—our cancer exists. Both the disease and its treatment can affect our physical capabilities, and it can be life-shortening.

Reality—we experience a wide range of emotions. We may begin with shock and denial, experience anxiety, fear, and stress, demonstrate anger, sadness, and defensiveness, exhibit symptoms of depression, and feel out-of-control and victimized. Each of these emotions may come and go over time in varying degrees. And important to acknowledge, each is normal.

Hope—we search for knowledge, adopt a future orientation and a desire to take action, and take advantage of our indomitable human spirit.

Hope—we acknowledge and appreciate the unrelenting dedication and progress of researchers, medical professionals, and the broader cancer community.

Hope—we build strength through the support of loved ones and through our personal brand of spirituality.

Balance—we accept reality and nurture hope as we mindfully create our support team, have crucial conversations with them, and with intention, develop meaningful and realistic plans for our future, both for the cancer part and the non-cancer parts of our lives. When diagnosed with cancer, we can either let the disease and its treatments happen to us and consume our lives, or we can be mindful about addressing both the disease and everything about our lives that is not the disease. This is certainly not to minimize the reality that is cancer and its treatments, but rather to attend to our lives in a way that helps make them the most they can be.

Early in his classic 1968 novel, *Cancer Ward*, Nobel Prize winner Aleksandr Solzhenitsyn, himself a cancer survivor, included two chapters to establish the perspectives of key characters. One chapter is entitled "The Patients' Worries" and the other is "The Doctors' Worries."

Like Solzhenitsyn, I believe that our relationship with cancer can be best understood through a multifaceted view of the disease. In that regard, let's explore a variety of perspectives that can become the basis of our life plan going forward. What are the experiences of those who have already interacted with the disease? What are their lessons learned? What actions did they take or not take? How did they cope with the inevitable emotions? How should all of this inform each of us who has been diagnosed or each of us who is a loved one of a cancer survivor? Answering these questions will help us in *Balancing Reality and Hope*.

So let's learn from others, take control of what we can, build our support systems, have the crucial conversations, and mindfully plan both parts of our lives—and let's do it together.

Alan Spector

In the spirit of preparing to build your cancer and non-cancer plans, which you'll do in the final two chapters, I'll prompt you at the end of the first seven chapters with some questions for you to answer for yourself. Take a moment to capture your thoughts on each question.

1. What are the three key ideas I learned from this chapter?
2. Based on what I learned in this chapter:
    a. What will I want to build into my plans?
    b. Who might help me do this?

Reality

"Reality has a way of intruding.
Reality eventually intrudes on everything."
Joe Biden

"Resilience is accepting your new reality,
even if it's less good than the one you had before."
Elizabeth Edwards

Reality is Stubborn

The late science fiction writer Philip K. Dick, many of whose novels and short stories have been adapted for film (such as *Blade Runner, Total Recall, Minority Report*), once described reality as that which, if you stop believing it, does not go away.

Reality is stubborn. No matter how hard we deny and fight it, it is what it is. A cancer diagnosis is exactly that. There may be a number of possible actions we can take in response to the diagnosis, but one of those choices is not, "Ignore it, and it will go away."

Guidance from Susan Sontag

In her 1978 essay, *Illness as Metaphor*, the late writer and political activist Susan Sontag, at the time a breast cancer survivor, maintained that no one who has been diagnosed should allow themselves to be distracted from an urgent quest for the best treatment for their illness.

I ascribe to her argument and am personally thankful to researchers, funders, and my medical team for developing and administering an effective care plan when I was diagnosed with Chronic Lymphocytic Leukemia (CLL) in 2010. My primary care physician urged prompt attention from a specialist to assess my elevated white blood cell count. The hematologist diagnosed the disease, described it to me in a way I could understand, and quickly got me on track with the best treatment approach.

Was it difficult, emotional, and disorienting to hear the diagnosis? Yes! Did I allow myself to be in denial? Definitely not! Did I educate myself about the disease and treatment options? Absolutely! Did I work with the oncologist to put the treatment regimen in place? Immediately! Did I look for other possibilities that would complement my treatment plan? Surely! No time for distraction; only for learning, decision making, and action.

I am in Sontag's camp in that there is grave risk in any vagueness of language or thinking that serves to detach a survivor from the reality. At a time when dealing with facts and taking timely and appropriate action is the order of business, any distraction that delays acknowledging a diagnosis and making urgent treatment decisions is dangerous.

In these first chapters, we'll address the reality of cancer head on. We'll explore what cancer is and begin to better understand what questions we should be asking and what actions we should consider taking. We'll do this, among other ways, by tapping into the experts, hearing stories of those who have gone before us, and extracting the lessons they've learned. This will help us, survivor and loved one alike, begin to envision what may be ahead of us as we transition from diagnosis to and through treatment, adjusting to the physical and emotional changes we'll experience throughout survivorship.

As I noted in the Introduction, throughout the book we'll use the term "survivor," sometimes interchangeably with "patient," according to the definition used by the National Cancer Institute of the National Institutes of Health: "a person is considered to be a survivor from the time of diagnosis until the end of life."

Chapter 1

Did You Know?

"I keep dreaming of a future, a future with a long and healthy life,
not lived in the shadow of cancer but in the light."
Patrick Swayze

"Yes, I have cancer and it might not go away,
but I can still have a future because life goes on."
Kris Carr

Bob Miller
"Game On!"

When he is not working out to build his strength and endurance for his competitive rowing passion, Bob Miller fills his retirement life with a diverse portfolio of meaningful activities. As a former corporate Human Resources executive, he applies what he learned during his career to his retirement roles as an Executive Coach and a Retirement Life Planning Coach.

Bob is also an active volunteer, frequent traveler, and proud grandfather. But it was his rowing that gave him the initial signals that something might be wrong. While training with his rowing partner in their quest to be Masters National age-group champions, which they successfully accomplished, Bob noticed pain across his shoulders and lower back. He first attributed the pain to an even-more-rigorous-than-normal training regimen and "never being this old before."

Bob got another signal while he was volunteering for Habitat for Humanity—he spiked a 102-degree fever. Several weeks later, Bob, who lives in Cincinnati, Ohio, was in a singles rowing competition in Toledo and feeling miserable, "as though I had weights hanging from my body." He finished a full minute behind his normal time. Over the following weeks, the incidents of pain, fever, and bouts of general malaise increased in frequency.

Acknowledging that the issues were a result of more than training and age, Bob went to his doctor, who guided him to specialists, who prescribed a number of tests, including a CT scan. Bob describes the scan results as having "lit the thing up." He was ultimately diagnosed with Follicular Lymphoma, a slowly-growing cancer of the lymphatic system and a subtype of non-Hodgkin Lymphoma.

His response to the diagnosis was mixed. He experienced relief for finally knowing what it was after many uncertain months, but, at the same time was thinking, "Oh, Shit! What does this mean and where do we go from here?" He uses the words "fear" and "dread" to further describe that moment.

But Bob knew he needed to learn, make decisions, and act. He dug into the data on-line, tried to filter out what seemed not to be credible, and formulated meaningful questions for his oncologist. Her response was to thank him for being, unlike many of her patients, calm, focused, and in a learning mode. She said, "I'm going to put everything in front of you," and literally pulled out her diagnosis book to share the details, including there being a 50 to 80% survival rate. Like most of us might do, Bob did the math and translated the stats into a 20 to 50% non-survival rate.

This early dialogue created an open, collaborative doctor-patient partnership to deal with the disease, and that relationship has stood the test of time. Bob values knowing the facts and understanding the reality, and his doctor values the license she has to be fully open with him.

Despite the quality of Bob's communication with his oncologist, he has heeded a friend's advice. This friend, who had been diagnosed about a year before, suggested that Bob take an audio recorder to each doctor's visit to make sure that in the midst of all of the shared facts and persistent emotion, he could revisit the conversation after the fact to make sure he really heard everything. Bob has followed the advice, but only after clearing it with the doctor.

Several years later and as of this writing, he is doing well and approaching his final maintenance chemotherapy session. And he has also gone on to win an International rowing championship in Copenhagen. You go, Bob! As you say about your approach to your cancer, as you say about life in general, and as you say about your rowing, "Game on!"

Cancer Windows

Although Bob Miller committed himself to learning as much about his cancer as possible, he could not literally see it. But wouldn't it be intriguing to be able to do so at its most fundamental level? Would you want to?

Fortunately, there are many who dedicate their lives to doing just that; finding ways to see the essence of cancer so as to profoundly understand how it works and to develop and deliver ever-more effective treatments. We'll meet and learn from many of these research professionals throughout the book, especially in Chapter 6.

As but one example, researchers in the Netherlands implanted a transparent material in the abdominal cavities of mice to enable viewing of the actual activity of cancer—observing cells as they settle to establish tumors and as they migrate to new organs. In her 2012 article, "A Window into Cancer" for *TheScientist* magazine, Sabrina Richards begins, "A literal window into the insides of mice is giving scientists a peek at the accumulation of cancer cells in organs deep within the body."

The researchers, Jacco van Rheenen, PhD and colleagues, refer to the technique as "intravital microscopy." A round surgically-implanted glass coverslip creates a window, enabling a new and different perspective on cancer to increase our collective understanding.

Although van Rheenen looked through real windows, most researchers look through metaphorical ones. We will as well, and in doing so, learn more about the disease, which in general, we call cancer. While researchers are seeking ever-more sophisticated views, we'll start with the basics.

Cancer—a Primer

Each survivor has a specific cancer diagnosis. It may be a type of lung or breast cancer, one of the blood or gastrointestinal cancers, or any one of the many other possibilities. You will want to learn as much as you can about your specific diagnosis to help you have the crucial conversations with your medical team and your loved ones and to help you fully participate in making good decisions about your course of treatment. That being said, there are some common things to know across all types of cancer.

The disease was first called "cancer" in about 400 BCE by Hippocrates, a Greek physician who has been referred to as the Father of Medicine. He called it "karkinos," which is Greek for crab. There is only speculation as to why he used the word. One theory is that tumors he was seeing were hard, like a crab's shell. Another is that the pain experienced by his patients caused by a malignant tumor reminded him of the sharp pinch of a crab's claw.

In 47 AD, a Greco-Roman philosopher, Celsus, although not a doctor, compiled an encyclopedia of medicine. He named the family of diseases "cancer," the Latin translation of "karkinos," the crab. About 100 years later, a physician named Galen further established the name, when he observed veins and tributaries emanating around the tumor mass. He commented that they reminded him of a crab's legs. For more than 2500 years, the disease has been recognized by Hippocrates' original designation, yet what we now know about cancer is obviously well beyond what the ancient Greeks and Romans could deduce or even imagine.

When all is normal, our body's cells grow and divide to form new cells that serve to fulfill any number of functions. When cells grow old or are damaged, they die off, making way for new cells. Cancers can be caused when some cells begin to divide abnormally, continue to do so, and spread to surrounding tissues. In other cases, old, damaged cells do not die off as they should.

The abnormalities in our normal cell division process occur at the genetic level. Most of these mutations are just random mistakes not cleansed by our immune system. A smaller percentage are inherited, and some can be caused by exposure to environmental cancer-causing elements (carcinogens).

In some cancers, this production of abnormal cells forms tumors, solid masses of tissue. If a tumor is malignant, its abnormal cells can migrate to nearby tissues and even throughout the body via the bloodstream or lymphatic system to form new tumors in other body sites. This is referred to as metastatic cancer. If the dispersed cancer cells are the same as those from the original location, the cancer that has spread is still referred to by the primary site. Breast cancer that has spread to the lung is not lung cancer, but rather metastatic breast cancer.

Some tumors are benign (not malignant), and although they will not spread and do not usually grow back when removed, they can still cause problems because of their size. Benign brain tumors, for example, can be life-threatening.

Other cancers, like the various types of leukemia, do not form tumors, but rather the abnormal cells crowd out the normal and necessary cells in the blood and bone marrow.

Cancer cells do not have the same characteristics of normal cells, which have specific functions throughout the body. When abnormal cells displace normal cells, those body functions can suffer. The cancer cells can also cause problems in that they can exhibit uncontrolled growth; they can disable the immune system to prevent it from protecting us from infections and other conditions; and they can actually protect themselves from our immune system.

Allow me to pause for a moment here to emphasize that this cancer primer and the information throughout the book is shared in the spirit I described in the "Introduction." Our mutual objective is to learn as much as we can about cancer in general and our cancer specifically, such that we can meaningfully participate in the development of our treatment plan. In that spirit, we'll be reviewing information that may not be easy to read and acknowledge, but it is the reality.

If you're interested in going beyond the basics of the primer, one good starting point is the annual progress report provided by the American Association for Cancer Research (AACR). It provides information about how cancer forms and how it is being combatted, including the latest progress.

Reality and Hope—Statistics

The late neurosurgeon, Dr. Paul Kalanithi, authored *When Breath Becomes Air* after being diagnosed with metastatic lung cancer. Kalanithi died at age 37 before his book was published. Throughout this book, we'll acknowledge some of his profound insights about his disease and about how to think of life as a survivor.

This first reference to Kalanithi helps us grasp cancer statistics. In his book, he recalled preparing for a conversation with a patient on whom he had operated for glioblastoma, a fast-growing malignant brain tumor.

"After surgery, we talked again, this time discussing chemo, radiation, and prognosis. By this point, I had learned a couple of basic rules. First, detailed statistics are for research halls, not hospital rooms. The standard statistic, the Kaplan-Meier curve, measures the number of patients surviving over time. It is the metric by which we gauge progress, by which we understand the ferocity of a disease. For glioblastoma, the curve drops sharply until only about 5 percent of patients are alive at two years. Second, it is important to be accurate, but you must leave some room for hope. Rather than saying: 'Median survival is eleven months' or 'You have a ninety-five percent chance of being dead in two years,' I'd say, 'Most patients live many months to a couple of years.' This was, to me, a more honest description. The problem is that you can't tell an individual patient where she sits on the curve. Will she die in six months or sixty?"

With Kalanithi's caveat in mind, let's still review some statistics to "gauge progress" and "understand the ferocity of the disease." As I noted in the "Introduction," when I looked out of the Siteman Cancer Center windows and observed the busy intersection in which I estimated there to be about 100 people in cars and on foot, about 40 of those people had already been or will be diagnosed with cancer in their lifetimes.

You can find more detailed data in the Appendix, but for perspective, here's an overview:

> ➤ The rate of cancer incidence is high and will continue to increase due to improvement in diagnostic capability and the aging of the population. About 600,000 cancer deaths occur in the U.S. every year. For direct medical costs alone, we spend about $80 billion in the U.S. annually. Sobering? Yes. Is the news all bad? Absolutely not.

> ➤ Despite an increased incidence rate since 1975, the mortality rate has dropped and continues to do so. Are these reasons to have hope? Yes. Is further progress expected? Absolutely!

> ➤ Statistics regarding childhood cancers, those among survivors under 15 years of age, tell a similar story. There are a significant number of diagnoses and deaths each year, yet survival rates have meaningfully improved and continue to do so. If you are reading this book as a loved one of a childhood survivor, your perspective and role are certainly different from those of adult survivors and loved ones. But you'll find the book's concepts applicable, and periodically you'll find specific reference to childhood cancer.

This overview and the statistics you'll find in the Appendix give us reason to balance reality and hope, but they are only in reference to the collective family of cancers and not each specific diagnosis; not yours and not mine. As did Bob Miller with his Follicular Lymphoma and as I with my Chronic Lymphocytic Leukemia, you can benefit from a deeper understanding of your particular cancer, thereby getting both the reality and the hope down to an intimately personal level. Doing so will enable you to intelligently collaborate with your medical team, build your structure of social and emotional support, and develop your life plan going forward.

There are a number of resources beyond your medical oncology team that can help you better understand both the essence of your cancer and options to address it. We'll address resources throughout the book, but for now, here are just some examples to give you an idea of the range of possibilities:

> ➤ American Cancer Society: a good place to start is their annual "Cancer Facts & Figures" publication
> ➤ Leukemia & Lymphoma Society: they have local chapters in many cities and a national "Information Specialists" call and chat capability (a great example of disease-specific support)
> ➤ Cancer Support Community: they have both a national "Cancer Support Helpline" and local affiliates in many communities
> ➤ WebMD: one of many credible on-line sites that contain significant information about specific diseases, symptoms, treatments, etc. (make sure of information integrity as you do your searches)
> ➤ National Council for Cancer Survivorship: they have a "Cancer Survivor Toolbox®" available on their web site

We'll also address the resources available for you to consider complementary and alternative approaches. Some swear by therapies in conjunction with, and some even instead of, the conventional medical standard-of-care and others strongly oppose these approaches. Because our general premise is that each of us owns the decision-making that will yield our cancer therapy plan, it should be helpful for you to think about how complementary and alternative approaches might or might not apply to you. We'll get into these approaches in more details later.

The Cancer Community

Certainly not by choice, but the reality is that you have become a member of the broader cancer community. But what does that mean, and where do you fit?

Let's start by looking at your cancer timeline. You were living your life cancer-free, or at least you didn't know you had cancer, and were likely not spending much time, if any, thinking about it. At some point, you may have developed symptoms that caused you to visit a doctor to investigate further. Recall Bob Miller's pains, fevers, and general feelings of weakness.

Or you may have been symptom free and discovered the possibility of cancer as part of a routine examination. Recall my annual physical that found white blood cell counts to be high with no symptoms to that point.

Whether you experienced symptoms or not, that pivotal doctor's visit during which you received your diagnosis introduced you to your local cancer community, with all that implies—additional doctors and their staffs, medical tests and the technicians who conduct them, treatment regimens and the experts who administer them, and your personal support systems. Although individuals may change over time, this community will accompany you on your transition throughout survivorship.

Although you are not likely to experience it directly, there is also a much broader cancer community, beyond your local team, that will have or has already had a meaningful effect on you.

There is a large and complex research community, professionals around the country and around the world, searching for a deeper understanding of cancer and seeking more effective prevention methods, detection techniques, and therapies. These same researchers then work with other medical professionals to translate the science into actual practice.

The treatments available to you today started in one or more labs many years before, were qualified by extensive and expensive clinical trials, scaled up to be available across geographies, and approved as the new standard of care for your particular cancer. We'll learn about the research community more extensively in Chapter 6.

Research and related activities require significant funding, and thankfully, there is part of the cancer community that generates the money, albeit not always sufficient to take full advantage of the science in a timely way. There are organizations who raise funds to fight specific cancers or cancer in general. Examples are the Leukemia & Lymphoma Society and the American Cancer Society, respectively. Cancer Centers also raise funds for their specific research programs. Examples are the Lombardi Cancer Center at Georgetown University, the Siteman Cancer Center in St. Louis, and the University of Colorado Cancer Center.

These organizations count on the generosity of donors who are dedicated to supporting research activities. Many of these donors are grateful patients, who have been helped by previous research, or the families of patients who have lost their battle with a specific cancer. We'll revisit these organizations and donors throughout the book and in more detail in Chapter 7.

Another segment of the cancer community was active well before each of us was diagnosed. These are the medical professionals who both tend to us and who educate and train future generations of oncologists and other specialists. And there are the organizations who make sure the medical facilities, such as hospitals, cancer centers, laboratories, administrative staff, and pharmacies are available when we need them.

So far, it is likely that the components of the cancer community have not surprised you, but there is one segment that may seem less obvious. It is the advocates—perhaps you know them better as lobbyists. While that term frequently carries negative baggage, let's look at what these dedicated people do in the cancer field.

Perhaps you have been diagnosed with cancer, but you struggle with having the financial means to afford the treatment you need. Perhaps you live in a remote part of your state, far from the best cancer centers. Perhaps you live in a medically underserved urban area. If you fit any of these scenarios or others like them, you may not have the "access" to the medical support you need and deserve.

Many organizations, as an example, Fight Colorectal Cancer, have advocacy programs that work at the national and state levels to educate legislators to affect public policy, funding, and legislation to help ensure access for everyone, regardless of demography or geography.

There is a significant business sector within the cancer community. We already mentioned hospitals, but there are also pharmaceutical companies, insurance companies, and many others that serve cancer patients in an effort to both fulfill needs and make a profit.

There is a governmental component. The National Cancer Institute of the National Institutes of Health, for example, allocates funding and sets the standards for cancer centers and research institutions. The Food and Drug Administration evaluates and monitors the efficacy and safety of therapies. There are other agencies at the federal, state, and local levels that are patches in the cancer community quilt.

And there is a component of the community referred to as alternative, complementary, functional, holistic, or integrative health approaches. This segment includes practitioners who offer non-conventional approaches that are frequently coordinated with conventional therapies. We'll delve into this in Chapter 3.

There are even more aspects of the cancer community, like support organizations, pastoral counselors, cancer coaches, and social workers. More about these and others throughout the book.

Does the community always work in a seamless, fully-integrated way? No. Is there opportunity to critique motives, actions, and results? Yes. But overall, does the community make progress? Again, yes. And to each of us, as the survivors for whom the community exists, that is a good thing.

Take a moment to capture your thoughts on each question—it will be helpful when you build your plans in the final two chapters.

1. What are the three key ideas I learned from this chapter?
2. Based on what I learned in this chapter:
    a. What will I want to build into my plans?
    b. Who might help me do this?

Chapter 2

Diagnosis

---

*"What I quickly learned after my diagnosis
is that the world of a cancer patient
has many parts and a good deal of uncertainty."*
Tom Brokaw

---

*"When you receive a cancer diagnosis,
you're more vulnerable than at any other time in your life."*
Suzanne Somers

Diagnosis is Good

Former Cincinnati Reds outfielder, Ken Griffey Sr., was diagnosed with prostate cancer at age 55, having been tested since his mid-30s. His mother made sure Griffey and his four brothers knew and acted on the importance of regular testing. She profoundly understood the consequences of her sons not being tested, because four of her brothers, Griffey's uncles, died of prostate cancer.

Knowing that a diagnosis is good, in respect to addressing the disease, Griffey says, "Men don't want to admit they have a [health] problem...But speaking up about questions or concerns can be the difference between early detection and not being around next Father's Day."

Not every cancer lends itself to regular testing that can lead to early detection—at least, not yet. And not every cancer has an answer—at least, not yet. But the principle is the same. If the cancer is there, diagnosis is good. Griffey, who is still doing well, would attest to that.

Don Pearline
More than His Fair Share

Don Pearline has had more than his fair share of cancer encounters.

His first wife, Carol, died of breast cancer and his brother of lung cancer. Don is a prostate cancer survivor. His most recent cancer confrontation was the loss of his 38-year old daughter, Rachel, to gastric cancer.

Prior to her death in late 2015, Dr. Rachel Pearline had completed a fellowship in oncology at the University of California-San Francisco, giving Rachel's survivorship and Don's experience as a loved one a very different perspective than that of most families touched by cancer.

While still in high school, Rachel was inspired by her mother's death to commit to a career in oncology. Along her path, besides receiving her MD from Tulane School of Medicine, Rachel earned her Master's in Public Health from the Tulane School of Tropical Medicine, completed her residency at NYU, ran marathons to raise money for cancer research at Memorial Sloan Kettering Cancer Center, made use of her fluency in Mandarin to study drug resistance in China, volunteered to help survivors being taken to New Jersey in the aftermath of 9/11, and helped provide medical care after Hurricane Katrina in New Orleans, at NYU's Medical Center after Hurricane Sandy, and after the Haiti earthquake.

Rachel had several surgeries to treat her cancer, including having her stomach completely removed. Through the ordeal, Rachel and Don received reasonably optimistic signals from physicians. Unfortunately, that did not last—Rachel's surgeon informed them that her condition had worsened, and there was nothing more that could be done.

Don's throat constricted and he had to sit down for fear of falling.

"It's scary," Don says, "it's not like a broken arm—set it and it will get better. With cancer, there is so much uncertainty. Will the treatment work? Is the cancer hiding somewhere else? Will the treatment work where it is targeted but not prevent metastases? These thoughts are persistent."

Yet Don is proud that his family members and he have all approached cancer with positive attitudes. They all did their best to make sure their lives and the lives of those around them could continue to be as normal as possible. Carol and Don, for example, wanted their daughters to experience their early teenage years without being too adversely affected by Carol's illness. And Rachel worked with her own cancer patients until a month before she passed away.

Rachel, from her perspective of both oncologist and patient, taught Don to think in terms of what she referred to as "integrative oncology." Along with her surgeries, Rachel also tried acupuncture, medical marijuana, and changing her diet to be more organic and minimally processed.

Becoming a master at confronting cancer is not something any of us want cast upon us. However, there is a lot to be learned from someone who has had more than his fair share of familial diagnoses. These are but a few of Don's lessons learned.

> ➤ As both a survivor and a loved one, "learn everything you can."
> ➤ Make use of every resource you can find—you never know where a meaningful suggestion will come from.
> ➤ Many people will have suggestions about what you should do—some may be good, but seek to understand their basis for the suggestion, then do the research.
> ➤ Be aggressive—advocate for what you know is right.
> ➤ "Go to the biggest, best-est, cancer treatment center you can."

Of note, since Rachel Pearline's death, the University of California-San Francisco has created an endowment in her name to support an annual fellowship, and she posthumously received the Annual Research Humanitarian Award.

Art or Act

Some of the words and phrases in the following definitions of "diagnosis" have the sound of certainty, while others less so.

> ➤ Merriam-Webster, "the art or act of identifying a disease from its signs and symptoms."
> ➤ Dictionary.com, "the process of determining by examination the nature and circumstances of a diseased condition."

> Oxford Learner's Dictionary, "the act of discovering or identifying the exact cause of an illness or a problem."
> MedicineNet.com, "the process of weighing the probability of one disease versus that of other diseases possibly accounting for a patient's illness." (MedicineNet.com's definition of "differential diagnosis")

Regardless of the definition to which you ascribe, the "art" or "act" of diagnosis is complex, bringing together your symptoms, your medical history, the results of a physical examination and tests, and the physician's expertise and experience.

Now that you or a loved one has a diagnosis, it would be worth going through a checklist, at least a mental one, but preferably written, to make sure you fully understand the diagnosis. Doing so will put you in good stead to actively participate in the critical decision-making you have in front of you.

Crucial Conversations

"It was impossible to get a good conversation going,
everybody was talking too much."
Yogi Berra

"Let us make a special effort to stop communicating with each other,
so we can have a conversation."
Mark Twain

Wait! What? On the surface, Mark Twain's statement almost sounds more like a Yogi-ism than one from the master himself. Yet just as Yogi's quotes always (well, almost always) have a deeper meaning, so do each of these Twain/Berra sayings. Each is an insight into the value of conversation in lieu of simply talking.

Our lives are filled with opportunities for meaningful conversations, but we don't always take advantage. There may be no time during which having crucial conversations is more important than through cancer survivorship.

Throughout the book, I'll alert you when we're going to address one of those crucial conversations. We'll start with this one between doctor and patient.

Oncologist : Patient

In her book, *What Patients Say, What Doctors Hear*, Danielle Ofri, MD, writes, "For all of the sophisticated diagnostic tools of modern medicine, the conversation between doctor and patient remains the primary diagnostic tool...the patient's verbal description of the problem and the doctor's questions about it are critical to an accurate diagnosis."

The value of a high-quality conversation between the oncologist and the patient begins during the first appointment and continues well beyond the diagnosis. This is a partnership in which each of the participants plays a vital ongoing role. Diagnoses need to be thoroughly understood, treatment plans need to be devised, agreed upon, and put in place, and adjustments need to be made based on changing circumstances.

Each conversation is critical, and thereby, the quality of contributions from each participant is critical. Unfortunately, that is frequently not the case. As an example, Dr. Ofri, despite the title of her book, also addresses what doctors say and what patients don't hear. She refers to studies that report how many patients are unaware of seemingly important aspects of their disease and its care. In one study, fewer than 50% of patients being discharged from a hospital could name their main diagnosis. When doctors were asked, more than three-quarters were confident their patients knew the diagnosis.

In the same study, of those being discharged, fewer than 20% could name their primary hospital doctor. When the doctors were asked, fully two-thirds were confident their patients knew their names.

From another study, Ofri reports, "Whether patients are leaving the hospital, the emergency room, or a regular office visit, less than half the information lobbed at them is typically retained."

Think about that for a moment. These are not casual chit-chat conversations with friends at a local coffee shop. In a situation where one's health is at stake, the conversation is less than 50% effective.

A more cancer-specific communications study was conducted jointly by the University of California, Davis and the University of Rochester. It focused on those with advanced cancer. Nearly 70% of patients believed they had a meaningfully better chance of two-year survival than did their doctors.

There is a lot going on here that makes a quality conversation difficult. Either party may be unskilled at expressing themselves or listening well. The emotions of both giving and hearing medical information may make it difficult to stay focused.

Doctors may be reluctant to be fully upfront with bad news. Perhaps as fellow human beings, it is simply difficult to tell someone they have a serious illness, let alone one that is terminal. Or as some doctors report, they are hesitant because of a concern that a dire prognosis will cause the patient to become withdrawn or depressed, inhibiting them from participating in their care.

In another section of her book, Dr. Ofri reports that it has been shown that after receiving bad medical news, a patient typically doesn't take in much of what follows. She also indicates that emotions may even get in the way of comprehension if the medical news is good.

Regardless of the issue that prevents a quality conversation, it's important for the patient to understand what has been said and that everything that needed to be said was, in fact, communicated.

One of the questions Dr. Bartlett, my oncologist, typically asks at my routine every-three-month visits is whether I have been feeling fatigued. Well yes, I worked out at the gym three days in a row, did some heavy-lifting landscaping at home, played in a night baseball game, and went out to a late dinner with friends. In addition I'm getting up a couple of times each night to go to the bathroom and don't always get back to sleep easily. And by the way, I am (as of this writing) 72 years old. Yes, sometimes I feel fatigued. But is the fatigue a result of my CLL or of all of the other things. Should I say yes or no? I opt for "No," assuming that if it was fatigue from the CLL or a remnant side effect of my chemotherapy, I'd know it when I felt it. But maybe I'm wrong. I may not be holding up my end of the conversation.

Learning from Ofri and to reemphasize the lesson we learned from Bob Miller in Chapter 1, it is frequently difficult to take in, understand, and remember all of the information that is coming your way. Some options that have helped others include taking copious notes yourself, recruiting an advocate, perhaps a family member or friend, to join you to listen and take notes, and/or to record the conversation with your doctor.

Despite the complexity of the communications, it is vital that the patient and loved ones hear and absorb all of the necessary information. To help you determine if everything has been covered, here is a list of questions you may want to consider asking your doctor. The questions are derived from a number of sources, including the National Cancer Institute of the National Institutes of Health, the American Cancer Society, the Mayo Clinic, and WebMD.

To ensure you get the information you need, it would be helpful to write down the questions you want to ask your doctor. During your appointment, first hear your doctor out. He or she will likely cover much of what you want to know. Then ask any remaining questions and request clarification where you need it. Be sure to leave with a level of understanding that satisfies you.

> ➢ What type of cancer do I have? You'll want to know both the general terms and any specifics that may differentiate it from others. For example, if you have lung cancer, is it squamous cell carcinoma, large cell carcinoma, or another? If you have leukemia, is it chronic lymphocytic (CLL), acute myeloid (AML), or another?

> ➢ What stage is my cancer? There are several systems that describe cancer stages—the most widely used has stages 0-to-IV. Although most cancers don't have a Stage 0, when they do, it indicates abnormal cells are present but there may be no other symptoms. The higher the number of the remaining stages indicates a tumor is larger and the cancer has spread, either to nearby tissues for the lower stages or to distant body parts at Stage IV. The stage of your cancer helps indicate the best treatment choices. To note, the stage of your cancer is indicated at diagnosis, and even if your cancer changes for the better or worse over time, it will continue to be referred to by its original stage designation.

> ➢ What is my prognosis? Decide how much you want to know about how serious your cancer is and your chances for survival. Knowing more can help with decisions you'll be making regarding medical or financial or relationship matters. Not knowing more may be right if the statistics and details will be confusing or unnecessarily frightening to you.

➢ How certain is the diagnosis? Depending on the answer, you may choose to seek additional opinions, or you may ask whether there are additional tests that are needed to become more certain. You may even want to do the research on your own to ask about specific tests that you deem appropriate.

➢ What are my treatment options and what do you recommend as the best course of action? And why? Will the treatment cure my cancer? If not, what can I expect the treatment to accomplish?

➢ What treatment side effects can I expect, and what can I do upfront to manage those effects? Should I expect pain and if so, what is available to help me cope with it? Said another way, what can I do to feel better before, during, and after my treatment?

➢ How can I access information about options for integrative oncology? Recognize that your doctor may only answer the questions about treatment options by dealing with conventional medical alternatives, which is fine but may not cover all the bases. You may also want to explore (and we'll address this in more detail later) non-conventional options, for example, nutrition, exercise, herbal remedies, stress management, and/or other lifestyle choices. You certainly can and should ask your doctor how to best access this support, but you may also need to search elsewhere to get the whole picture.

➢ When should I begin treatment? Will I be able to continue to work? How will treatment affect everyday living? Are there any restrictions I'll need to follow? Should I be concerned that the treatment or the cancer itself will make me infertile or impotent? The answers to these questions will help you make the necessary plans going forward.

➢ How can I learn about and access clinical trials that apply to me? We'll learn more about clinical trials in Chapter 6, when we address what the research community does and how they do it.

➢ How will we know if the treatment is working? What is the backup plan if it is not? The answers may involve additional tests. My first round of chemotherapy was successful as measured by blood tests, a bone marrow biopsy, and a physical examination, but I knew, because I asked, that there was an oral CLL medication approved if the chemo had not worked.

> ➤ Should I see a specialist? Or perhaps more than one? Your oncologist may very well be the right person to lead the medical care, but it would be helpful to know if there are other doctors who may be more skilled and experienced at addressing your particular diagnosis.

> ➤ Is there another cancer center that has a reputation for best addressing my particular cancer? If so, should I be going there? Why or why not?

> ➤ How does my cancer and its treatment interact with my other health issues? Make sure each of your doctors is fully aware of all of your medical issues and medications, and ask about interactions of each. In a perfect world, there would be one lead doctor who pulls your personal care physician, oncologist, and specialists together to make sure your care is coordinated. The reality is that such a circumstance is rare, so it behooves each of us to act, as best we can, as our own care coordinator or to have a loved one play that role.

> ➤ Who can best help me understand the cost and insurance implications of my cancer and its treatment? Depending on your particular circumstances, a cancer diagnosis can be financially challenging for the survivor and/or the caregiver. Some refer to this as "financial toxicity." It is best to get this question posed as early as possible to make sure you can get ahead of any planning and decision-making needs. Regardless of your financial circumstances, you should ask for the resources you need to ensure you are receiving the best care.

> ➤ What additional learning material do you recommend? Which web sites are credible? Your learning journey begins at diagnosis. Much of your information will come directly from your doctor, but your time with him or her may be limited. You can use research materials to learn more and to formulate key questions for your next doctor visit.

> ➤ What are the logistics of my treatment? It may sound trivial, but you want to get the details right on all counts. What is the date and time, starting and ending, for each treatment? If I'll be there through meals, should/can I bring food? Where will I be treated? Do I need someone to accompany me? Where and how do I register

when I get there? What documentation do I need to bring with me? What happens if I miss a treatment? Who do I call if I have problems between appointments, and what symptoms should I report immediately? Don't be bashful about making sure you can envision the treatment process—although the doctor and nurse have been through this many times, it's likely your first time.

Some of us are more comfortable than others with asking a lot of questions. Some of us are more comfortable than others with what we are willing to hear about our diagnosis and prognosis. It is certainly a personal decision about how much you want to ask and know. That being said, even if you are less comfortable with the process, I'd suggest you stretch yourself toward asking more versus less to at least see how it works for you.

Ludmila and Lindsay

Ludmila's story takes place in 1955; Lindsay's in 2016.

Ludmila was in her 50's; Lindsay was 33.

Ludmila worked in a hospital in Soviet Central Asia; Lindsay worked in Midwestern America.

Ludmila is a fictional character we meet in Aleksandr Solzhenitsyn's novel, *Cancer Ward*; Lindsay is real, and we learn about her in a blog post.

How different they are, yet how connected they are, both to each other and to each of us.

Ludmila and Lindsay are both oncology medical professionals, doctor and nurse, respectively. Both were diagnosed with advanced-stage cancer. Both realized that despite dealing with cancer survivors on a daily basis for years, they did not fully relate to what the patients were going through emotionally.

Ludmila

In *Cancer Ward*, Ludmila Afanasyevna Dontsova is the clinical staff doctor in charge of radiotherapy and fluoroscopy. After we learn Ludmila has cancer and has likely waited much too long to address her symptoms,

Solzhenitsyn, at the time a cancer survivor himself, opens a chapter aptly entitled "The Other Side of the Coin,"

> *Dontsova had never imagined that something she knew inside and out and so thoroughly could change to the point where it became entirely new and unfamiliar. For thirty years she had been dealing with other people's illnesses, and for a good twenty she had sat in front of the X-ray screen. She had read the screen, read the film, read the distorted, imploring eyes of her patients. She had compared what she saw with books and analyses, written articles and argued with colleagues and patients. During this time what she had worked out empirically for herself had become more and more indisputable, while in her mind medical theory grew increasingly coherent. Etiology, pathogenesis, symptoms, diagnosis, the course of the disease, treatment, prevention, prognosis—all these were real enough. The doctor might have sympathy for the patient's resistance, doubts and fears; these were understandable human weaknesses, but they didn't count for anything when it came to deciding which method should be used. There was no place left for such feelings in the squares of logic.*
>
> *Until now all human bodies had been built identically as described in the standard anatomy text. The physiology of the vital processes and the physiology of sensations were uniform as well. Everything that was normal or deviated from the norm was explained in logical terms by authoritative manuals.*
>
> *Then suddenly, within a few days, her own body had fallen out of this great, orderly system. It had struck hard earth and was now like a hopeless sack crammed with organs—organs which might at any moment be seized with pain and cry out.*
>
> *Within a few days everything had been turned inside out. Her body was, as before, composed of parts she knew well, but the whole was unknown and frightening.*

Lindsay

On November 14, 2016, just weeks after being diagnosed with stage III colorectal cancer and about to begin chemotherapy and radiation to be followed by surgery, Lindsay Norris, an oncology nurse, posted a blog entitled, "Dear every cancer patient I ever took care of, I'm sorry. I didn't get it."

Lindsay's post is more extensive, but here is a representative paragraph that lines up with Ludmila's experience.

> *I didn't get what it felt like to actually hear the words. I've been in on countless diagnoses conversations and even had to give the news myself on plenty of occasions, but being the person the doctor is talking about is surreal. You were trying to listen to the details and pay attention, but really you just wanted to keep a straight face for as long as it took to maybe ask one appropriate question and get the heck out of there fast. You probably went home and broke down under the weight of what you had just been told. You probably sat in silence and disbelief for hours until you had to go pretend everything was fine at work or wherever because you didn't have any details yet and wanted to keep it private still. You probably didn't even know where to start and your mind went straight to very dark places. That day was the worst. I'm sorry. I didn't get it.*

Vincent

Lindsay Norris and Aleksandr Solzhenitsyn's Ludmila teach us that the emotions of a diagnosis are normal and frequently misunderstood. Here's another example.

Among the most credentialed oncologists in the world is Vincent DeVita, Jr., MD He is credited with developing a cure for Hodgkin's lymphoma via combination chemotherapy, and DeVita has been the Director of the National Cancer Institute and the National Cancer Program, Physician-in-Chief at Memorial Sloan Kettering Cancer Center, Director of the Yale Cancer Center,

Professor of Medicine, Epidemiology, and Public Health at the Yale School of Medicine, and President of the American Cancer Society.

In 2006, he was diagnosed with a fast-growing form of prostate cancer. In a chapter of his book, *The Death of Cancer,* DeVita describes his journey of diagnosis to treatment to remission. Among the phrases he uses are the following:

"...I lived in a daze."

"My deepest fear..."

"I was shocked."

"Paralyzed by anxiety..."

"...disengaging my mind from the worry."

"Every time the anxiety surfaced..."

"I was overcome with relief..."

"...the worry seems to seep in before each test."

Have you experienced feelings like these since you or your loved one received the diagnosis? Are you still feeling them? The emotions are normal. The evidence needs go no farther than the DeVita example. Despite profoundly understanding the science, he was still subject to the kinds of feelings we all have. He wrote, "You might assume with my background...that I wouldn't be bowled over, to the point of numbness, by my diagnosis. But you would be wrong."

Tom

Perhaps Tom Brokaw is best known for the 20+ years he spent, beginning in 1982, as the anchor and managing editor of the *NBC Nightly News.* He has also hosted NBC's *Today Show* and, for a brief time, *Meet the Press.* He is a prolific author, including his much-acclaimed book, *The Greatest Generation.*

In 2013, at age 73, Brokaw, who was still very active in the broadcast industry, in his literary career, with his family, and in his passion for the outdoors, was diagnosed with multiple myeloma, a blood cancer of the plasma cells. His survivorship prompted him to author *A Lucky Life Interrupted: A Memoir of Hope.* Among his insights relating to the diagnosis, he writes, "For all the attention cancer receives publicly, such as at

Stand Up To Cancer events during the World Series, or when big tough NFL linemen show up in pink shoes to draw attention to breast cancer, my guess is that most of us duck it by thinking, Not me."

Of being tested at the Mayo Clinic, Brokaw writes, "A new clock was ticking in my life and I didn't have a clue. In about thirty minutes I went from the illusion of being forever young to the reality that life has a way of choosing its own course."

Brokaw's wife of a half-century was not with him on his Mayo Clinic trip, and he waited to tell her about the diagnosis until they were face-to-face, "I had rehearsed what I was going to say because I wanted to be precise but also because I was struggling to deal with that strange tug-of-war between my new reality and a way of life I couldn't quite believe was slipping away. I said nothing about dying from it, because I didn't expect to, but I said, 'This will change our lives.'"

Ludmila, Lindsay, Vincent, Tom, each survivor, each loved one, you, and I have been compelled to deal with two things—the reality of the disease and the reality of the emotions triggered by the diagnosis.

Crucial Conversation Alert

Who to Tell?

One of the early crucial conversations you will have is telling people about your diagnosis. But before you have those conversations, you need to determine who you will and will not tell.

There is no prescribed best answer for everyone. Because each of our circumstances is different, this is a very personal decision. Here are some examples from which you might begin building your pluses and minuses of informing just a few or communicating broadly.

Tom Brokaw used a "bad back" story to explain his visible multiple myeloma issues, so as to not need to share broadly that he had cancer. In his book, he helped describe his struggle to determine who to tell and not tell, "Several close pals were worried I was hiding something very serious. We were part of the circle of Nora Ephron, the essayist, playwright, screenwriter, director, social arbiter, and den mother for a range of friends uniformly in awe of and in love with her. When she kept her rare form of leukemia secret until the week she died we were at once bereft and acutely conscious of what we don't know about our closest friends."

Nora Ephron's sister, author, screenwriter, playwright, and producer Delia Ephron, was diagnosed at age 72 with Acute Myeloid Leukemia, AML, the same disease Nora died of. Delia was given access to a promising, but not yet FDA-approved drug. About this she wrote, "I felt grateful for that, but I wished so much that this drug or something suited to Nora had existed when she was sick. I was lonely for her, more than ever."

She followed with thoughts about choosing who to tell, "Like my sister, I started lying. I told lots of lies to people I love. To people I work with. About why the screenplay wasn't in, why I had to miss appointments. I'm a terrible liar. I said whatever came to my head. I even borrowed a friend's eye disease. All I could think was, if I tell one person and they tell another, my news would be public, published as: 'Her sister died, she's dying, too.'"

Bob Miller, the follicular lymphoma survivor you met in Chapter 1, chose to share broadly, using CaringBridge.org, for two reasons. He wanted to proactively "manage the message" to make sure accurate and timely information was available, and he felt, which turned out to be right, that the outpouring of support that followed helped both him and his loved ones.

In an AgingCare.com blog post, Betsy Hnath, whose husband is a stage IV metastatic melanoma survivor, relates her struggles soon after his diagnosis. Being his caregiver and rearing a two-year old at the same time was difficult enough, but she also had to deal with their decision "to keep things very private." They told only immediate family and very few friends.

She writes of George's severe treatment side effects and her steep learning curve, "I was brand new to caring for anyone in that kind of need...Fear and anxiety began taking over my mind and body, and I struggled to find the appropriate place and time to allow the growing swell of my inner emotions crack through. I began experiencing panic attacks, and without anyone to talk to about what was happening while enduring a long Maine winter, I was trapped."

Building support for the caregiver may be a reason to share the diagnosis more broadly.

By the way, Hnath is herself a stage II breast cancer survivor, a fact she shares openly.

Although most people tell those closest to them, a UK study indicates that about 25% of cancer survivors consider even keeping news of their diagnosis from family and close friends, and the primary reason is to protect loved ones from worrying. That is certainly one consideration, but there are many more as well.

The examples above and guidance from organizations like the Leukemia & Lymphoma Society and the American Cancer Society prompt these questions that may help you determine who to tell. There are no right or wrong answers to these questions, but your answers may be useful to you.

> Are you concerned about whether your cancer will define who you are to others?
> Do you want to or need to expand your support system?
> Do you feel you want to have a broad group of people with whom you can talk openly about your cancer?
> Are there visible indicators of your cancer such that people will know/suspect anyway?
> Do you want to control your message as did Bob Miller?
> What concerns do you have about how colleagues and your boss will react at work?
> What concerns do you have about how other people will react to the news and how they might treat you differently?
> Do you live away from immediate family?
> Do you want to give others the opportunity to openly express their fears and hopes?
> Do you want to make sure your close family and friends who are providing your caregiving have the support they need, unlike Betsy Hnath's situation?

Grieving

It is not uncommon for us to think about grief primarily in the context of the death of someone close to us. Yet in a June 4, 2013 blog post, "The Best Grief Definition You Will Find," Russell Friedman, coauthor (with John W. James) of *The Grief Recovery Handbook*, engages us with a broader understanding of grief and asserts that the most basic definition is "the normal and natural emotional reaction to loss or change of any kind."

Being diagnosed with cancer is just that, a major loss and change. Before diagnosis, we were living a cancer-free life. It may have been a life with which we were satisfied or one with which we were not. Regardless, that life had some structure and predictability. We had routines, relationships, plans, aspirations.

Irrespective of the type of cancer, the stage, or the prognosis, our diagnosis is life-changing—grieving and the emotions that come with it are inevitable. Each survivor and each loved one will experience a wide range of emotions that will ebb and flow. How and how long we experience them will vary for each of us.

Friedman makes the point, based on his extensive study of grief and on helping many cope with it, that the cliché applies, "Everyone grieves in their own way and at their own pace."

One of the realities I highlight in the book's "Introduction" is "we may begin with shock and denial, experience anxiety, fear, and stress, demonstrate anger, sadness, and defensiveness, exhibit symptoms of depression, and feel out-of-control and victimized."

The diagnosis is real—the emotions are real—the grieving is real.

Jill Chapin
"Breathtaking"

Jill Chapin is an author, columnist, and activist who can teach us a lot about responding to a diagnosis. She wrote this essay after her daughter was diagnosed with stage II breast cancer.

Two weeks shy of her 28th birthday and the birth of her first child, my daughter discovered a malignant lump in her breast. I can most accurately describe my reaction to that news as simply breathtaking, but not in the grand way that word implies. I mean it in a quite literal sense, as in the taking away of one's breath, as in a body slam, as in a sucking out of all oxygen in the room.

What kind of sick joke could place side by side the most joyous occasion in one's life with news like this? How could one phone call separate my entire life into two parts - the "before the call" and "after the call?"

And just what is the protocol here for revealing one's emotions? How could I appear so down at the moment of my grandchild's birth, or so up when my daughter is overwrought with her own health issues? The truth is I felt both ways, probably at the wrong times, but I was too confused to cope with the etiquette of inappropriate emoting.

Prior to this sharp turn in my life, I've always had to rely on an empathetic nature and a vivid imagination in understanding the sorrows of others. Because, as unlikely as it seems, I've always been lucky. I guess I've known it since I was a child and could spot four-leaf clovers as easily as my friends could find bright yellow dandelions. I always wondered why I never experienced really bad things. As the decades wore on, I wondered if I would be able to handle "real life" when it would inevitably catch up with me.

Now I know. When your luck seems to have run out, you simply deal. You not only adjust and adapt, you also find yourself literally making deals with yourself, making up any kind of imaginary trade-off to make this all go away.

But life goes on and we are all doing fine, really. Armed with information forged from a ride on a steep learning curve, a plan of action, a sensitive and savvy team of caregivers, plus a wealth of the best kind of family and friends, in many ways, we are truly in a better emotional place than before. And of course, my husband and I are enchanted with our new granddaughter.

But those who know me best see a subtle change that is best expressed in a fortune cookie I once read. It said that sudden misfortune does not change people; it merely exposes them. Now I have been exposed to my daughter as I really am - selfish and greedy. Selfish because when I bought into this All-I-Want-Is-A-Healthy-Baby mantra, I meant my baby. And greedy because - as unstable as this may seem - the one thing I want more than anything in this whole world is cancer. But I don't want just any old cancer.

I want hers.

Seek Help

Although diagnosis-triggered emotions are normal, we are affected by them in different ways. Some of us may experience psychological symptoms that require professional help.

In 2012, a study of over 10,000 cancer patients was reported in the *Journal of Affective Disorders*. In the study, 19 percent and 13 percent showed clinical levels of anxiety and depression, respectively. Another 23 percent and 17 percent reported subclinical anxiety and depression symptoms, respectively.

Many cancer treatment facilities have begun to screen for these issues and have resources to help address them. If you are concerned that you or a loved one is falling into this area of concern, seek the help you need.

Take a moment to capture your thoughts for this chapter.

1. What are the three key ideas I learned from this chapter?
2. Based on what I learned in this chapter:
   a. What will I want to build into my plans?
   b. Who might help me do this?

Chapter 3

Treatment

"Cancer is a scary thing, and you have to deal with it seriously."
Kareem Abdul-Jabbar

"Scars are tattoos with better stories."
Anonymous

The Pod

Whenever I check in for an appointment for a blood test, for other procedures, or for an infusion session, there sits an invariably helpful and congenial registrar, "Name and date of birth, please."

I have gotten to the point, and you probably have or will as well, where I now lead with that information, not giving the registrar time to ask. It's as if my date of birth is an actual extension of my name—Alan Spector May 20 1946.

Did you hear the one about the newly-diagnosed cancer patient who is settled in for his first chemotherapy infusion? His wife, his chemo-buddy for the day, joins him about an hour later. The patient greets her and gleefully says, "The nurse keeps asking me for my date of birth. I think she's going to get me something."

By the way, why is it that when the registrars, nurses, and other staff first greet you, they frequently ask the question, "How are you?"

I understand it's used as a generic greeting, but I always want to answer, but never do, "That's what I'm here to find out" or "I have cancer, how do you think I am?"

Remember Grumpy, one of the Seven Dwarfs? I don't want to be that guy. It wouldn't help anything, and the staff is just being welcoming and nice. So, "I'm fine, thank you, how are you?"

One view through the blood lab waiting room windows at the Siteman Cancer Center is of downtown St. Louis and the Gateway Arch. The windows let in the light and comforting warmth of the morning sun. At the cancer center, comfort is a good thing.

There are other windows in view from the comfortable seats of the waiting room, where some of the chairs are recliners for those who need and deserve an extra dose of comfort. There is, for example, a glass partition between the lab waiting room and the waiting room I will be moving to next, that of my oncologist. The glass allows me to observe the constant flow of patients, caregivers, nurses, and other staff. It is a very busy place—and busy means there's a lot of cancer.

The infusion rooms, sometimes called pods, where chemotherapies, blood transfusions, and other therapies are administered, have windows to the outside. Light is plentiful; light is needed.

Perhaps as telling as where the windows are is where they are not. They are conspicuous by their absence in exam rooms and rooms in which procedures such as CT scans and bone marrow biopsies are performed. It is apparent and appropriate that there are no windows in those places where privacy is so important.

Speaking of privacy, what about the infusion pods? Should those not also be places of discretion? They are anything but that. And I've concluded from personal experience that it's just fine that they are not.

My first infusion was on September 3, 2014. In my regular three-month checkup appointment a few weeks earlier, Dr. Bartlett got right down to it, "We've been monitoring your rising white blood cell count and other factors for several years, and it's now time for treatment. There are three indicators. First, your white cell count is doubling at close to every six months. Second, your recent bone marrow biopsy shows a very high percentage of CLL cells. Finally, your creatinine level is not out of range but is at the high end—earlier treatment will help ensure no reduction in kidney function."

"OK," I respond, knowing that this time would eventually come, "What happens next?"

I sat in my reclining chair in the infusion pod, hooked up to my hanging therapy cocktail of Rituximab and Bendamustine, fed to me intravenously by a pump through plastic tubing and into my arm through the IV catheter that had been inserted and taped to me to make sure it stayed put.

In the pod with me were nine other patients, seven in recliners like mine and two in beds. Each of us was offered warmed blankets, which I quickly learned to accept—there's that comfort thing again. And each of us is surrounded by visitor's chairs, a small TV on an adjustable gantry, a small side table, a retractable curtain, and most importantly, the infusion gear, rigged to a pole on wheels—pumps, tubing, hooks for hanging the bags of medications or blood or whatever is to be infused. There are electrical outlets and ports in the wall for oxygen and who knows what else.

We are also surrounded by the sounds of the pod, two of which are most prevalent. One is the constant chatter of patients, visitors, and staff. This quickly becomes background noise and doesn't feel intrusive, with a few exceptions. The other is the occasional beeping of the infusion pumps. It doesn't take long to figure out what it means when a pump rhythmically beeps, calling to the attention of the nursing staff that an infusion bag is running low or a tube has become crimped.

I become aware of the metaphorical windows between my life and the lives of the other survivors in the pod, between my treatment and theirs, between my thoughts and theirs. There are also metaphorical windows between the nurse's station and me, between the volunteers, one who is a high-school classmate I swear to secrecy, and me, between the custodians and me. I am looking through each of these windows. Are those on the other side looking back?

The IV catheter is in my arm, having been inserted as soon as I was settled in my chair. Others arrive with permanent IV ports in their chests to facilitate more frequent infusions.

I make one observation very early in my first session. Every patient thanks every nurse, staff member, and volunteer for every big or little thing that the person does for them. There are plenty of thanks to give out, and every one of them seems sincere. I know mine are.

Several patients appear well—either their cancer is working invisibly inside of them, or they are legitimately on the mend. I suppose I appear well with the possible exception of the enlarged lymph node on the right side of my neck. Fortunately, the node is significantly smaller than it was just a month ago, when it appeared to be golf-ball size. Some research led me to a report of a successful Phase II clinical trial of high doses of green tea extract helping CLL survivors. I have been taking these morning and night, and Dr.

Bartlett agrees that my nodes had been reducing in size, even before the chemo, and that I could continue to take the extract.

Other patients in the pod do not appear well at all.

Young Man

I peer through one metaphorical window at a young man with a knit cap on his hairless head. He is reclining in one of the beds. He is 32 years old—I know this because before the nurses hang his treatment bags, they do the standard quality assurance test to confirm the right medication is going to the right patient. He states his name and date-of-birth.

During the day, he receives both chemotherapy and a blood transfusion. In many ways, I can tell this is one of a long series of such sessions for him. When he returns from wheeling his IV pole to the bathroom, he is familiar enough with the equipment to plug it back into the wall himself before getting back in bed.

He speaks with a slight accent, which I ascribe to rural Missouri. It is not uncommon for survivors within a cancer center's catchment area (the area the center serves) to travel for treatment.

The young man is quick to laugh as he interacts with the two women who are visiting with him, but between the laughter, time spent reading on his tablet, and munching on snacks from a bag, he is prone to long bouts of staring blankly into space.

We learn through the not-so-private conversation that the women have been trained to administer chemotherapy to him at home. They seem confident.

Nicknames

I help pass the time by assigning nicknames that seem to suit my pod mates, but which I would never say out loud.

I peer through a metaphorical window at Edgy Earl, who sports a large cover over one of his ears. The contraption looks like half of a wrestling headgear held on by a sweatband, all white. He is wearing a Chicago Bears sweat suit on his short squat frame and is distinguished by a large bushy goatee that seems to be tolerating chemo better than his very thinning white hair. He is visited by a resident and is visibly and audibly upset that the visitor is not "the" doctor. His wife is working hard to keep him calm, but nobody in the room blames him for being on edge. He will soon have a first or a subsequent surgery on his ear.

I peer through a window at Mario. When the big guy enters the pod, accompanied by his wife and son, he is jovial. He is assigned to one of the beds, but it looks like the only reason is that a chair is not available. He takes off his shoes, gets into bed, and immediately falls asleep. The nurse awakens him to put in his IV, and he can't get back to sleep. Jovial Mario becomes Grumpy.

I peer through a window at Rosie. She is thin, but it does not seem to be from the disease or the treatment. Her hair is also thin, and that very much seems to be the result of previous treatments. A bandana is attempting to cover her head. Rosie is in the recliner immediately to my right. Her platelet count is extremely low. Her doctor has ordered a transfusion.

I peer through a window at Poor Fred. Fred is 58 years old, concerned about dying, and wanting to talk about it. He has lost his hair, but his gray moustache is in full bloom. The only time he stops talking about dying during the first hour is when he is snacking, which is actually most of the time. When it is time to put in his IV, it becomes quite a scene. The nurse cannot find a vein, and Poor Fred is suffering. The nurse finally calls in another to try and luckily, mostly for Poor Fred, but for the rest of us as well, the second nurse is successful. To everyone's delight, Poor Fred sleeps through most of the remainder of his session.

I peer through a window at Pained Paula. A very large woman on oxygen is wheel-chaired into the pod by her daughter. Paula can barely walk from the wheelchair to her lounger. She wants a bed, but one is not available. Paula is negotiating, with appropriate advocacy by her daughter, with the nurses to give her pain meds to allow her to tolerate sitting for a long time. One nurse leaves the room, apparently to find out if they can provide the meds, and returns to inject them into the woman's IV. During all of this, the daughter knowingly attaches Paula's oxygen to the wall outlet. Shortly thereafter, the chemo fluids are hung. Pained Paula never gets comfortable.

I peer through a window at Loud Guy. Big boisterous blue-collar type walks in and greets every nurse, aid, custodian, and volunteer by name. As he moves through the pod to his chair, he introduces himself to each of the other patients. His name is Lloyd, which I translate to Loud. But it becomes abundantly clear that Loud Guy has a large heart. A curtain is pulled around his chair so the nurses can access the port in his chest. We can hear the conversation—one of the nurses is saying she can't wait until payday on Friday. Loud Guy sincerely offers to front her food and gas money, which she declines.

Bart

I have no idea why I think of him as Bart. He is one of the few in the pod whose real name I don't hear. Just as with all of the others, I only view this circumstantial acquaintance through the metaphorical window between us. I really don't know Bart, but I sense that he needs someone to know him. He has no visitors and I surmise that he never does.

Bart's age is indeterminate. He looks 80, but like one of those people who is not really that old. Late 50s? 60s? He is gaunt, but the word does not really do the trick. Picture the photos of a very tired Abraham Lincoln during the most difficult times of the Civil War, but with even less humor in his eyes.

Bart has either been at this infusion thing for a long time or he was diagnosed late in the progression of the disease.

He is staring at the ceiling, mouth slightly open, breathing with apparent difficulty. What could he be thinking? What would I be thinking? I know what I am thinking, and I am in significantly better shape than he.

The Good News

A number of the questions for your doctor listed in Chapter 2 are intended to help develop your treatment plan.

> What are my treatment options and what do you recommend as the best course of action? And why? Will the treatment cure my cancer? If not, what can I expect the treatment to accomplish?

> What side effects can I expect, and what can I do upfront to mitigate those effects? Should I expect pain and if so, what is available to

manage it? Said another way, what can I do to feel better before, during, and after my treatment?

➢ When should I begin treatment? Will I be able to continue to work? How will treatment affect everyday living? Are there any restrictions I'll need to follow?

➢ How will we know if the treatment is working? What is the backup plan if it is not?

The good news is that you own your health and wellbeing and have the opportunity to fully participate in and be the ultimate decision-maker in your treatment plan. In doing so, you likely have two primary objectives. One is to achieve the best possible results regarding the cancer itself, whether it be cure, remission, or an increased chance or length of survival. A second is to experience the best possible quality of life in both the near and longer term.

In the vast majority of cases, your treatment plan will be the conventional medicine standard of care combined with a supportive care plan.

But what does that mean, and how do those terms compare to others you may have heard; for example, complementary, alternative, and palliative?

Terminology

The next several sections address the different approaches to therapy. These can be confusing, because of the plethora of terms in use, some of which are used interchangeably, sometimes inappropriately. Before getting into more details on each, here are the key terms, what they mean, and how we'll use them.

➢ Conventional Medicine: approved treatments available to medical professionals that include both the standard of care and promising therapies in clinical trials. These may include, for example, chemotherapy, immunotherapy, surgery, and radiation. Conventional medicine is also referred to as mainstream, orthodox, or Western medicine.

You will likely find sources in which conventional medicine is also referred to as traditional medicine. At issue, however, is that others who administer and follow ancient healing philosophies refer to them as, among other terms, traditional Chinese medicine. To avoid this confusion, I'll not use the word traditional. If you hear it from someone, make sure you know to what they are referring.

➢ Supportive Care: support provided by medical professionals and other disciplines that is coordinated with your oncology team to prevent and relieve the symptoms and stress of the cancer and its treatment for both the survivor and loved ones. This may include, for example, psychiatric support, nutritional guidance, and stress management counseling. It can be provided prior to, along with, and/or after conventional therapy. At times, supportive care is referred to as and used interchangeably with "palliative care."

➢ Complementary Health Approach: similar to supportive care, this addresses the symptoms and stress of cancer and its treatment; however, it is provided by practitioners who may not be in coordination with the medical oncologists. This may include, for example, yoga, massage, and spirituality practices. You may also see this referred to as holistic, functional, lifestyle, or integrative medicine. As the term implies and as we'll use it, this approach is complementary to conventional medicine therapies.

Although you'll frequently see this referred to as "complementary medicine," the National Center for Complementary and Integrative Health of the National Institutes of Health employs the term "health approaches" instead of "medicine," so we will as well.

➢ Alternative Health Approach: similar to the complementary health approach with one key exception—when the practices are used in lieu of and not in concert with conventional medicine therapies.

Conventional Medicine

These evidence-based treatments are grounded on the results of scientific research, are in wide use, and are the accepted arsenal of options your oncologist has at his or her disposal. For any specific diagnosis, this includes what is referred to as the "standard of care," which has been demonstrated by the research and medical communities to be the currently best known therapy and approved for use.

Your diagnosis, which includes identification of your specific cancer, its stage, and your prognosis, is the basis for which one or a combination of the conventional medicine categories of treatment are right for your doctor to recommend and for you to consider.

> ➤ Chemotherapy: drugs that can be taken orally, by injection or infusion, or applied to the skin for the purpose of killing cancer cells or stopping them from dividing
>
> ➤ Immunotherapy: substances used to enable the body's own immune system to fight the cancer
>
> ➤ Surgery: a procedure to remove a cancerous growth or to explore an area to learn more about the extent of the cancer
>
> ➤ Radiation: a high-energy source applied to kill cancer cells and shrink tumors. It can be administered by an external beam, by radioactive material called "seeds" placed near cancer cells, or by an oral or IV-fed radioactive substance that reaches a tumor via the bloodstream
>
> ➤ Targeted Therapy: drugs used to identify specific types of cancer cells and kill them with less harm to normal cells than other therapies (sometimes referred to as "precision therapy")
>
> ➤ Hormone Therapy: substances targeted to block the body's natural hormones, which may be enabling the cancer

Supportive Care

It is a reality that a combination of your symptoms and treatment side effects may become difficult to cope with physically, emotionally, practically, and spiritually. This is where supportive care comes into play.

Your supportive care team may include your oncologist, his or her staff, a pain specialist, specially-trained nurses, social workers, clergy, a nutritionist, physical and occupational therapists, a grief and bereavement counselor, volunteer visitors, or a child life specialist, depending on your needs. This team of professionals may work together as an integrated unit or individuals may work independently with you.

The team may be helpful in mitigating your cancer or treatment symptoms, such as pain, nausea, and fatigue. They may help you understand your diagnosis and treatment options. They may support your emotional, social, and spiritual needs. They may provide support for loved ones. And they may provide support for what may be practical challenges you face, such as managing your finances, dealing with insurance, ensuring you have needed transportation, or setting up your home to accommodate your physical needs.

Survivors and their loved ones may not always take full advantage of supportive care for a number of reasons. They may inappropriately equate it with hospice care and thereby wait too long, perhaps until the survivor is sicker or the family is under greater stress. We'll look at hospice care in more detail in Chapter 8.

They may believe that supportive care is not available during the active administration of conventional therapies, yet it can start as soon as the diagnosis is made and continue throughout and beyond the period of treatment.

Or they may hear it referred to only as palliative care and not understand the term. A study reported in 2013 by R. M. Maciasz, et al at the University of Pittsburgh found the term "Supportive Care" helped survivors and families better understand what was available versus "Palliative Care." As but one example, when patients were asked to describe the two terms, 51% responded, "I don't know" for palliative care, while only 1% did so for supportive care. Although the medical community still frequently uses the term palliative care, that may be changing. In Chapter 4, you'll meet Laura Melton, PhD, who leads a group at the University of Colorado Cancer Center called "Supportive Oncology."

Be clear with your oncologist about your needs and talk to him or her about how you can best meet them. He or she may be able to help directly or may refer you to someone else on your supportive care team.

"I Don't Know"

You'll also get to know John Marshall, MD in more depth in Chapter 4. He's an impressively credentialed researcher and global leader in the fight against colon and other gastrointestinal cancers. Marshall also has an active clinical practice.

He focuses appointments with his patients on helping them make informed decisions about their treatment plans, including introducing them, if they are eligible, to clinical trials. It is not uncommon, however, for patients to ask Dr. Marshall about complementary or alternative health approaches, everything from acupuncture to herbal supplements, from yoga to nutrition, from exercise to prayer, from enemas to hypnosis. Many of these questions begin something like, "My Uncle Charlie told me to try..." and end with, "What do you think?"

Marshall knows that many doctors do not condone these health approaches and let their patients know that in no uncertain terms. And he knows that some doctors include complementary approaches in their practices.

He chooses to respond with three messages, the first being, "I don't know." This nonjudgmental statement makes it clear that the non-conventional approaches are outside of his expertise and also intimates that not only does he not know, but many of these approaches have not been sufficiently demonstrated to be an effective standard of care. So, in essence, he would argue that nobody knows.

He follows up with, "If you think something will work for you, then it might help." The key words here are "think" and "might," as there can be a positive effect even if the patient only has an expectation that something will work. This is often referred to as the "placebo effect" (more about this later in the chapter).

Marshall's third message addresses a risk associated with the choice of a non-conventional approach. He tells his patients, "If you choose an alternative, let me know, so I can assess whether it may interfere with the standard treatment we've decided upon."

Although he does not say so explicitly, an inference in Marshall's third message is focused on "the standard treatment we've decided upon." If his patient chooses an alternative health approach to the exclusion of or delay in beginning the conventional medicine standard of care, he identifies another risk—the cancer may have that much more time to grow and spread if the alternative approach doesn't work.

Choices to Make

You have some choices to make; some may be in full consultation with your oncologist, some not. Do I work with my oncologist to incorporate supportive care? Do I look into complementary health approaches on my own? Do I consider an alternative health approach in lieu of conventional medicine?

Certainly, bring these choices up with your oncologist, but also be prepared to investigate them through other channels. Use every available credible resource to fully understand the risks and benefits.

You may elect to pursue one or more of these approaches. Recall Rachel Pearline, the oncologist who died of gastric cancer at age 38. Her knowledge and experience prompted her to complement conventional therapies to help manage side effects with acupuncture, medical marijuana, and a diet of more organic and minimally processed foods.

Each complementary option must be evaluated for its benefits and risks. But if an approach helps manage your symptoms and side effects, even as the result of the placebo effect, and it doesn't interfere with the efficacy of your conventional standard-of-care treatment, it might be right for you. If you choose to utilize a complementary health approach, follow Dr. Marshall's advice to let your oncologist know, so that he or she can assess the possible interactive effects with your conventional therapy plan.

Instead, you may elect to follow an alternative health approach. In their book, *You Did What?—Saying "No" to Conventional Cancer Treatment*, Hollie and Patrick Quinn describe their journey following Hollie's stage II breast cancer diagnosis at age 28. After surgery to remove her tumor, they opted to pursue traditional Chinese medicine and other lifestyle health approaches in lieu of chemotherapy and radiation, the conventional standard of care that was indicated for Hollie. The Quinns did the research on their own to confidently make this decision. As the title, *You Did What?*, implies, theirs was and remains a controversial choice among many, especially medical professionals.

There's another point of view from which to consider the practices included in a complementary or alternative health approach - that of someone without cancer. Perhaps you are a loved one of a survivor, or perhaps you are reading this book simply for interest. If so, consider this. Examples of these practices are proper nutrition, exercise, stress reduction techniques, and spirituality. These can make a difference in quality of life, whether you have cancer or not, and they are steps that can be taken to lower cancer risk.

There are other non-conventional health approaches that are less obvious—there is even laughter yoga. Khevin Barnes, a stage magician, certified laughter yoga instructor, and cancer survivor, makes it clear that he is not laughing at cancer but in spite of it. He then points out that this yoga practice "...is designed to encourage people to breathe properly. Deep breathing has been shown to lower blood pressure, reduce stress, diminish cortisol (the stress hormone), and more."

At a time when it may be difficult to absorb all of the information coming your way and to initiate a credible search for your full range of options, that is exactly what you need to do. We'll review later what resources may be available to help you through this difficult decision-making period, and we'll work together to build your team—a team that might include supportive care specialists and practitioners of non-conventional health approaches.

Placebo Effect and Attitude

If your doctor gave you a pill that had no active ingredient, like a sugar pill, and authoritatively told you it was a stimulant, would you expect your pulse rate and blood pressure to increase? How about having your reaction time improve? What if your doctor gave you the same pill and told you it would help you sleep, would you expect it to do so?

That's exactly what happened in a study of what is called the placebo effect. There is a link between mind and body, and the more strongly you expect results from a pill, a procedure, an injection, or other approach, the more likely those results will occur.

To be clear—placebos can't cure cancer, but the research consistently shows they can bring relief from symptoms like nausea, fatigue, pain, and anxiety.

Placebos also carry some risk. If someone follows an unproven treatment that acts as a placebo to gain some temporary benefit, they may convince themselves to continue to delay conventional therapy or choose not to have it at all.

Another risk is that the positive effects from a placebo may fade over time. You may be experiencing benefits from a complementary health approach, for example, that loses effectiveness. By the way, don't worry if you believe that the approach is working because of the placebo effect. Studies have shown that even when people know they are taking a placebo, doing so may still work.

Yet another risk is that some people experience negative side effects from the placebo itself. This phenomenon is sometimes referred to as the "nocebo effect."

Dr. Ofri believes the research about the power of attitude based on experience with her own patients. She writes, "...I also try to frame things as optimistically as possible, within reason. I don't want to be a Pollyanna or paint unrealistic expectations for treatments that offer little value. But if we've chosen a path of treatment together, I try to invest both of our expectations in the right direction. Our communications might be a bit of placebo, but if it can help without causing side effects, then it seems like a legitimate medical intervention to pursue."

Since we are dealing with reality in this section of the book, let's be real. It is unrealistic to be a cancer survivor or loved one and constantly have a positive attitude. The normal emotions of a cancer diagnosis include fear, anxiety, and sadness. It is possible that you feel guilty about experiencing these emotions, which may further add to your burden. Again, all of this is normal, and it flies in the face of an expectation of always staying positive.

It is also part of our reality that the research has found no correlation between positive attitude and any difference in the progression of cancer— unless, of course, a negative attitude gets in the way of following a treatment protocol.

But remember that you may have that second objective we talked about earlier-improving your quality of life, regardless of your prognosis. That's where attitude can come in, as it has been shown to make a positive difference in coping with both physical and emotional symptoms.

Placebo effect and attitude—cure? No. Quality of life? Yes.

Take Your Medicine

Regardless of the treatment plan you choose, one of its key success factors will be whether or not you adhere to the plan. For example, if you are monitoring your blood counts every three months, there is a risk if you miss an appointment. Or if you are taking daily medication to lower the risk that your cancer will return, it will be less effective if you neglect to take your pills.

The National Center for Biotechnology Information (NCBI) is part the National Library of Medicine, a branch of the National Institutes for Health. NCBI reports, "In some disease conditions, more than 40% of patients sustain significant risks by misunderstanding, forgetting, or ignoring healthcare advice."

Further, NCBI notes, "...nonadherence is also a risk factor for a variety of subsequent poor health outcomes, including as many as 125,000 deaths each year" and "estimates of hospitalization costs due to medication nonadherence are as high as $12.25 billion annually in the U.S. alone."

The risk of non-adherence is one of the many reasons to fully understand the details of your cancer diagnosis and your treatment options. If you make your choice of treatments based on an understanding of why they work, you are more likely to adhere to your regimen.

The medical community used to refer to this topic as "compliance," but that word implied a system whereby the role of the physician is to determine the right course of action, and the patient's job is to merely comply. "Adherence" is meant to more directly reflect a system in which the patient takes active ownership of his or her own healthcare decisions.

There are various reasons patients do not adhere to their plan. One is that the side effects of treatment can be debilitating. If this is the case for you, it might be the impetus to investigate a complementary health approach. As but one example, you may experience nausea with some treatments that deter you from staying the course. If so, there may be ways to adjust your diet, some people benefit from acupuncture or relaxation techniques, or your doctor might prescribe anti-nausea medications.

Several other reasons for non-adherence may interact with each other and be difficult to differentiate. You may become depressed, experience a lack of motivation, and/or feel profound fatigue. These can result from the cancer itself or from a treatment side effect. Be open with your doctor or nurse or perhaps a social worker about what you are experiencing, so they can help you find the right resources to address the issues.

If your treatment plan includes daily medications, you may be finding it difficult to remember to take your doses—maybe life's busy-ness is getting in the way. Consider keeping a medication diary that sits in a place you can't miss it—perhaps near your toothbrush, where you go after every meal. Consider an alarm on your watch, cell phone, computer, or even your pill bottle. Use a day-by-day pill organizer. If there is someone you see or talk to every day, recruit them as a medication buddy to ask you whether you've taken your daily dose.

If your issue is financial, ask your doctor, nurse, or social worker to help you identify possible resources to help you access the therapies you need. Some of the resources are hospital based, others reside in your local social services community, while others may be governmentally based. Manufacturers of oncology drugs usually offer financial assistance for expensive oral medications, and several independent foundations offer copayment assistance for treatment of many types of cancer.

Just as your course of therapy is a choice, so is adherence. If something is getting in the way, deal with it. Take your medicine.

Abandonment

Good news—for many cancer survivors, there will come a time when treatment is complete and progress is positive. This may also be a time when the frequency of doctor visits for regular monitoring can be reduced.

My brother-in-law, Harvey Ferdman, is a 15+ year colorectal cancer survivor. He once told me that there was a period in his cancer experience when he struggled with feelings of abandonment. I thought he was referring to being abandoned by friends and family who may have become skittish about Harvey's cancer. But I knew Harvey was surrounded by love and support, so his statement surprised me.

Then he explained that the abandonment was what he felt when his oncologist reduced his appointment frequency. After years of regular and intense sessions, Harvey had come to rely on the attention and support, and he rued losing that. He knew intellectually that fewer appointments was a good sign, but he could not avoid the feeling of neglect.

In his Cancer.Net article, "3 Tips for Transitioning Out of Cancer Treatment," Doug Mackenzie, a squamous cell carcinoma survivor, referred to the phenomenon as "care withdrawal." He wrote, "Six chemotherapy treatments and 37 radiation therapy treatments later, I was cancer-free. But I soon found that transitioning back into a normal routine was not easy."

His three tips:

1. Be prepared for care withdrawal. You will have formed unique bonds with your health care team during treatment, and you may miss the interactions and support that came with that.
2. Be aware of possible ongoing side effects. Although you have been looking forward to life-after-treatment, your "new normal" may include managing long-term effects.
3. Hold on to your social support. Your support system during treatment can also help you cope with any post-treatment issues.

Since Harvey made me aware of the abandonment issue, I've come across this concern in a number of references, like Mackenzie's. And as I've checked it with other survivors, I've gotten a knowing smile and nod. You may have a similar reaction—it's another one of those normal emotions.

By the way, there are two other uses of the term "abandonment" in the cancer literature. One is, in fact, when friends and family distance themselves from the survivor for any number of reasons. Let's hope this doesn't happen to us.

The other is when survivors abandon their treatment regimen. This is the ultimate adherence issue, frequently resulting from cancer's financial challenges. As noted earlier, if this is an issue for you, seek help to find resources. Dr. Harold Freeman, an oncology surgeon for 25 years at Harlem Hospital and former National President of the American Cancer Society among his many credentials, was interviewed on CBS. During the segment, he asked the rhetorical question, "Should poverty be an offense punished by death?"

In summary of these first three chapters, the cancer is real, the side effects of treatment are real, the emotions are real. It's incumbent on both survivor and loved ones to acknowledge the reality and, as difficult as it may be, to deal with it head on. Doing so is a good first step in *Balancing Reality and Hope.*

Take a moment to capture your thoughts for this chapter.

1. What are the three key ideas I learned from this chapter?
2. Based on what I learned in this chapter:
    a. What will I want to build into my plans?
    b. Who might help me do this?

Hope

"For when hope does awaken, an entire life awakens along with it."
John S. Dunne

"Hope is being able to see that there is light despite all the darkness."
Desmond Tutu

Genuine Belief

In his book, *The Anatomy of Hope: How People Prevail in the Face of Illness*, oncologist Dr. Jerome Groopman writes, "Hope, I have come to believe, is as vital to our lives as the very oxygen that we breathe." He adds, "Clear-eyed hope gives us the courage to confront our circumstances and the capacity to surmount them. For all my patients, hope, true hope, has proved as important as any medication I might prescribe or any procedure I might perform."

Studies support Dr. Groopman's observations, in that they have discovered correlations between the level of hope and a reduction of depression and anxiety, increased longevity, and an increase in pain tolerance.

That being said, I'm confident Groopman would not opt for hope in lieu of the best therapy plan. This is not about choosing treatment *or* hope—it's about choosing treatment *and* hope. It works in both directions. Understanding, deciding on, and committing to your treatment plan are actions that foster hope, and studies have shown that hope can enhance the efficacy of a treatment plan.

But what is "true hope," and how do we build it? It's important that we address these questions, because, as Groopman asserts, as the evidence grows, and as many of us intuitively sense, hope can be a key ingredient in our wellbeing.

Elizabeth J. Clark, PhD, MSW is the right person to get us started on understanding what hope is. She has been, among many other things, CEO of the National Association of Social Workers, Executive Vice President and COO of a grassroots organizing campaign by the National Coalition for Cancer Survivorship (NCCS) called "The March...Coming Together to Conquer Cancer," Chair of the Patient Access Committee of the Leukemia & Lymphoma Society Board of Directors, and Chair of the Board of Directors of the National Hospice Foundation. And she is the author of the book *Choose Hope (Always Choose Hope).*

In 1995, Clark wrote the first of what would become four editions of *You Have a Right to be Hopeful*, a publication of NCCS, the oldest survivor-led cancer advocacy organization. Clark sets the stage for her passion for this subject when she writes that the publication is, "Dedicated with love to my sister Eleanor, a twelve-year survivor of multiple myeloma. She well understood the importance of hope."

Thus, based on her personal experience and a long-studied point of view, Clark asserts her belief in the importance of hope, "For the individual and for the family, cancer has a profound negative impact, yet hopefulness and a positive future orientation are important components for quality of life in cancer survivorship."

Clark then begins to address the complexity of the concept of hope by referring to but a sampling of definitions. In short, these varied descriptions refer to hope as a way of feeling, thinking, and behaving; the desire for personal survival and the ability to exert a degree of influence; a means of coping by avoiding despair and making stress bearable; the combination of driving toward a goal and finding a way to reach that goal.

In addition, Clark posits, "...hope is a prerequisite for action."

While I agree, I would suggest that action is also a prerequisite for hope. Hope is not wishful thinking, which is merely passive. It is not Pollyanna optimism. It is not false hope, which does not acknowledge there will be roadblocks along the way. And hope is not the blind denial of reality. Rather, the sweet spot is *Balancing Reality and Hope.*

I would suggest that hope is taking action to develop the genuine belief that the future will be better than the present and/or better than should be expected.

As we've noted, each of our diagnoses is different. Each cancer, stage, and prognosis is different. The aspects of our life circumstances, base level of health and fitness, financial situation, access to health care, and the breadth and depth of our support system are different. And our fundamental predisposition for being hopeful is different.

Hope will vary over time. We may be dealing with pain. We may be suffering the side effects of treatment. We may get the news that a period of remission has ended. We may get the news that our cancer will be life-shortening. These are each possible realities, and each will make it more difficult to have hope. That being said, hope is possible, virtually regardless of our condition.

Herth Hope

Kay Herth, PhD, RN provides an additional perspective of how we can think about hope. She is Dean Emerita of the Minnesota State University Mankato's College of Allied Health & Nursing, and in 2011, she was inducted into the International Nurse Researcher Hall of Fame. Herth is an international expert on hope among people with chronic or life-limiting illnesses.

Her many contributions include the development of survey instruments that have been translated into multiple languages and used worldwide to measure a person's level of hope. Participants are asked to read a number of statements and decide whether "Never," "Seldom," "Sometimes," or "Often" applies to them for each statement. The overall hope level is determined through a scoring mechanism applied across all of the answers.

Consider these statements, extracted from Herth's surveys, as to how they further describe hope and to how they may apply to you.

> - I have a positive outlook toward life.
> - I have short and/or long range goals.
> - I can see possibilities in the midst of difficulties.
> - I have faith that gives me comfort.
> - I have deep inner strength.
> - I am able to give and receive caring/love.

> ➢ I have a sense of direction.
> ➢ I believe that each day has potential.
> ➢ I feel my life has value and worth.

A 2007 study in London used the Herth Hope Index to determine how the level of hope for cancer patients changes over time. The study included one group of patients being treated for their cancer and another group only on palliative care. The study indicated that the level of hope was not different, regardless of prognosis, across the two groups.

Hopefulness is conceivable, almost regardless of circumstance. This returns us to the question of how to build hope. How do we get to that "genuine belief that the future will be better than the present and/or better than should be expected?"

Making Hope Happen

The late psychologist Shane Lopez, PhD, senior scientist for Gallup and author of *Making Hope Happen: Create the Future You Want for Yourself and Others*, wrote, "our relationship with the future determines how well we live today."

I trust that Lopez would have approved that I use his book title for this section. He knew the importance of hope and reflected Groopman's view when he wrote, "hope is like oxygen."

Perhaps Lopez distilled his most encouraging insights, derived from years of rigorous research, into a single message, when he wrote,

- o *Hope matters*
- o *Hope is a choice*
- o *Hope can be learned*
- o *Hope can be shared with others*

To paraphrase Lopez in our context, *Balancing Reality and Hope* is crucial, and we can choose to make plans and take action to make our lives the best they can be.

Perhaps no one exemplifies this more than Teri Griege, author of *Powered by Hope* and president and founder of the non-profit by the same name. In 2009, Griege was diagnosed with stage IV colon cancer and given a dire prognosis. As a long-time endurance athlete, she had had a dream of competing in the Ironman World Championship in Hawaii. While still undergoing chemotherapy, Griege continued to train and in 2011, completed the Ironman, one of the great endurance challenges on the planet.

Since then, she has raced in all of the World Marathon Majors, and importantly, through her Powered by Hope Foundation, Griege demonstrates Lopez's principle that "Hope can be shared with others." Her definition of hope is "making the most of every day," and she refers to hope by her acronym, "How Ordinary People Endure."

Hope is something we can build, both as individuals and in partnership with loved ones and others in our support system. With that in mind, let's focus on "making hope happen" for each of us.

Building on the works of Groopman, Clark, Herth, Lopez, Griege, and others, we are able to identify the components of building hope. Recognize that much of what we have been doing together so far and what we'll be doing in upcoming chapters is following these steps.

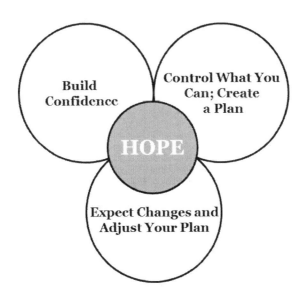

Build Confidence

One dictionary definition of "confidence" is "a feeling of self-assurance arising from one's appreciation of one's own abilities or qualities."

It would follow that building confidence would help ensure we feel empowered to make decisions and take actions that will positively affect our future—in other words, to build hope.

Regardless of your level of personal confidence in your pre-diagnosis life, it would not be unusual for you to lose confidence in the uncertainty and complexity that is cancer. What would it take to rebuild your life confidence as a survivor or loved one? Three suggestions:

1. Expand your knowledge about both your particular cancer and about the broader cancer community. Knowing as much as you can about your situation will enable you to confidently partner with your medical team and others to make the best decisions for you. Knowing more about the cancer community, understanding how research works and how to access clinical trials for newly developing therapies, and learning how to access support groups and other resources will all build confidence and hope. We'll address all of these and more.

2. Get to know your medical team both as professionals and individuals. The deeper your relationship and the deeper the crucial conversations you have with them, the deeper your confidence and hope will be. In the next chapter, we'll gain a broader perspective about the medical professional segment of the cancer community.

3. Explore your spirituality. Whether your belief system has a basis in organized religion or you approach this aspect of your life in a personal way, it can be a powerful component of building your confidence. Many U.S. medical schools now include courses about the relationship of religion and spirituality to health, and a vast majority of physicians believe spirituality can help healing.

As Shane Lopez wrote, hope helps "us see pathways where others see brick walls;" helps us "persevere when others give up;" and helps us "work harder when it would be easier to quit." It takes confidence to act this way, and building confidence builds hope.

Control What You Can; Create a Plan

Even before we were diagnosed, we knew that we could not control everything about our lives—a key to success was to identify things we could control and focus on those. The same is true post-diagnosis. Making decisions about and taking action on things we can control enable us to live in the moment with hope, knowing we are positively leaning into our future.

These are several key things we can control with a future-oriented approach:

1. Build a support team that is designed to help make the future the best it can be. We'll explore this in Chapter 8.

2. Have the crucial conversations with members of that support team, your loved ones, medical staff, pastoral counselors, and others about future plans, expectations, and hope.

3. Mindfully create a life plan for both the cancer and non-cancer parts of your life. Developing and living these plans will bring together everything we've discussed throughout the book. That's why the final two chapters will guide you through your personalized planning.

Expect Changes and Make Adjustments

What separates true hope from simply practicing wishful thinking is the expectation and acceptance that life circumstances change. The path to achieving our goals and dreams is often fraught with unanticipated roadblocks, but changes can be positive as well. In either case, when life's ups and downs occur, it may be time to alter your plan.

A former work colleague frequently said, "A plan is only something from which to deviate." He was not arguing against having a plan. On the contrary. He was arguing that having a plan is invaluable, because it is a foundation from which to respond to changing circumstances.

Accepting change and being resilient in response build hope.

Hope Horizon

One of the realities of cancer is that it may shorten our lives. Depending on our particular cancer, its stage, and the success of our treatment plan, we may die of the disease, live with it as a chronic condition, or be fortunate to be cured. I think we can agree that hope is important in any case.

Each of us, whether we have been diagnosed with cancer or not, has a "hope horizon" that informs us as to how far out in time we should be planning. For most of us, the hope horizon is uncertain, but there are some realities to heed.

It is a reality that my hope horizon at age 72, as of this writing, is shorter than when I was 35, irrespective of cancer. It is a reality that my hope horizon may be shorter because of my CLL. It is a reality that my hope horizon is longer because the cancer community developed effective therapies that were available when I needed them.

Consider what Lucy Kalanithi, MD wrote in her "Epilogue" for her late husband's book about his cancer experience, *When Breath Becomes Air*.

> *Relying on his own strength and the support of his family and community, Paul faced each stage of his illness with grace—not with bravado or misguided faith that he would "overcome" or "beat" cancer but with an authenticity that allowed him to grieve the loss of the future he had planned and forge a new one. He cried on the day he was diagnosed. He cried while looking at a drawing we kept on the bathroom mirror that said, "I want to spend all of the rest of my days here with you." He cried on his last day in the operating room. He let himself be open and vulnerable, let himself be comforted. Even while terminally ill, Paul was fully alive; despite physical collapse, he remained vigorous, open, full of hope not for an unlikely cure but for days that were full of purpose and meaning.*

A short hope horizon? Yes. But hopeful nevertheless? Yes. "Days full of purpose and meaning?" Absolutely.

Sweet Spot

Winnie the Pooh asked his friend, Piglet, "What day is it?"

"It's today," responded Piglet.

"My favorite day," said Pooh.

One doesn't need to be Winnie the Pooh or a Buddhist to know there is great value to living in the moment, neither dwelling on the past nor fretting what might or might not happen in the future. Yet we have been talking about leaning into our future. The magic is in balancing these two concepts.

Shane Lopez referred to the "Sweet Spot of Hope," describing it as "our thinking about the future overlaps with our thoughts about what needs to happen today. In the sweet spot, we believe in our ability to make the future better than the present, while at the same time we recognize the limits of our control."

Live in the present? Yes. Lean into your future? Yes. Build hope? Absolutely. Find the sweet spot.

Chapter 4

How Can We Help?
Medical Professionals

"As a cancer doctor, I'm looking forward to being out of a job."
Daniel Kraft

*"It is reasonable to expect the doctor to recognize that science
may not have all the answers to problems of health and healing."*
Norman Cousins

What Do You Do for Fun?

John Marshall, MD, is Chief, Division of Hematology-Oncology of Medstar Georgetown University Hospital and Professor of Medicine and Oncology, Lombardi Comprehensive Cancer Center. He is also Founding Director of the Otto J. Ruesch Center for the Cure of Gastrointestinal Cancer, a fitting position given his global leadership in the research and development of therapies for colon and other GI cancers, including being the principle investigator of over 150 clinical trials.

In concert with his commitment to his leadership roles and his research, Marshall maintains an active practice, seeing about 40 patients each week. He is perfectly suited to help us think about the criticality of, some of the issues in, and a physician's perspective about the doctor-patient relationship.

Marshall views his role with each patient as five-fold:

➤ Diagnose or confirm the diagnosis of the disease
➤ Educate the patient about the disease and its treatment options
➤ Understand the patient's desires
➤ Decide, with the patient, on the best treatment plan
➤ Expose eligible patients to clinical trial opportunities

Marshall observes that there are some common themes among his patients. They have, especially in early sessions, put their lives on hold until they figure out what's going on—they "have hit a wall." He describes them as typically being afraid and showing the signs of dealing with what may be the most stressful time in their lives. They are lost until he helps them develop an understanding of their situation and a strategy and plan for treatment.

Another common theme, he observes, is that most patients have a difficult time absorbing all of the information. In that regard, he urges patients to have an advocate to help listen to and understand what is being said. He encourages copious notetaking by both patient and advocate, and he is perfectly comfortable with having doctor-patient discussions recorded. Marshall knows it's critical to the effectiveness of future conversations, to treatment decision-making, and importantly, to the adherence to treatment regimens for patients to fully understand their situation and the implications of their choices.

There are differences among patients as well, especially as it relates to their level of knowledge and desire to learn. He finds some patients do their research, tapping into their "net-village" (Marshall's term for a personal network), diving into credible on-line resources, and reading everything they can get their hands on. Others either don't have the resources to do this self-learning, are paralyzed by their situation such that they can't take initiative, or are fundamentally afraid of what they might learn.

Marshall also finds some patients wanting to know the details of their prognosis, while others simply want to be told what the treatment plan is and to not have what could be a difficult and frightening discussion.

And he is blunt when he states his preference for patients who can fully participate in the development of their best care plan, "It's always nice when I have a patient who has at least a basic understanding of their disease."

To get to know his patients even better, Marshall asks a question that puts them off balance in a way that gets them to open up. He says, "I know we're here to talk about cancer, but what do you do for fun?" The conversation that ensues among his patient, the loved one in the room, and him helps Marshall get to know what's important to the patient and to the loved one.

The late neurosurgeon, Paul Kalanithi, revealed insights that parallel Marshall's experience and approach. He wrote, "Doctors in highly charged fields met patients at inflected moments, the most authentic moments, where life and identity were under threat; their duty included learning what made that particular patient's life worth living, and planning to save those things if possible—or to allow peace of death if not. Such power required deep responsibility..."

Depending on his patient's situation, Marshall may probe further to learn what the patient desires as a basis for jointly developing the best treatment plan. Marshall might ask, "How long do you want to live?"

The response is typically a number many years out from the patient's current age. Marshall then follows up with a quality-of-life conversation, asking something like, "What if you were incontinent, requiring 24-hour care, and didn't know who you were?"

One way for a survivor or loved one to further deepen the discussion is to ask, "Now that you know my diagnosis and you know me better, if your mother or spouse or dear friend were in my situation, what would you advise them?"

These conversations are complex, difficult, and crucial, all at the same time, but they help doctor and patient frame the treatment strategy and plan going forward.

Trust

Rick Boulay, MD, is Chief of the Division of Gynecologic Oncology at Lehigh Valley Health Network. His wife and father are both cancer survivors. In his article in the summer 2017 edition of *cure* magazine entitled "An Exercise in Trust: An oncologist considers the basis of the trust he and his patients share," he writes, "I think the doctor-patient relationship is sacred space. It defies definition or measurement. And in this space I am my best self. The idealized version of me. Judgment, preconception and blame are left outside the door. There is no room for that here. In this intimate space, honesty, transparency, and mutual respect quickly form the basis for a deep and trusting relationship like no other.

"...We will converse about the hopes and expectations you have...And when no more can be done to manage your illness and death is nigh, we will decide how best to manage your last few days or weeks on this earth with quality of life, as you define it, being our only goal."

Boulay seems to be a doctor who fully understands *Balancing Reality and Hope.* You may want to ask yourself, "Is it the kind of relationship I want to nurture with my doctor?"

The Best at the Best

First thing tomorrow morning, there is a survivor who has an appointment with the world's best oncologist for his or her particular cancer. Wouldn't you want that someone to be you? Why would you not want to be seeing the world expert at the cancer center with the world's best reputation?

That survivor may or may not be you or me. What we do want is to be seeing an oncologist who will ensure we get the right care at a cancer center that will professionally and compassionately deliver our required treatment.

Right doctor? Right place? What criteria would you use to determine the answers to these questions? Your doctor's track record? His or her bedside manner? Relative to Dr. Boulay's message, have you developed a trust relationship? The cancer center's reputation? Do they treat your kind of cancer on a regular basis? Access to clinical trials? Financial impact? Proximity to home? Some of these criteria or others may mean a lot or a little to you, or perhaps nothing at all.

Part of building hope is building confidence, a part of which is getting to know your medical team. As difficult as it may be, if you're not confident in or comfortable with your oncologist or your cancer center and you have the wherewithal to change either or both, do so. This is about your health, and you come first.

Other Docs

Hope can also derive from knowing that your medical team includes everyone it needs to. Recall one of the questions to ask your oncologist is, "Should I see a specialist, or perhaps more than one?"

Your oncologist may very well be the right person to coordinate your medical care, but it would be helpful to know if there are other doctors who are more skilled and experienced at addressing your particular diagnosis and needs. Or there may be other physicians who can provide a second opinion if desired.

In addition to your primary oncologist, some of the other docs who are ready to step forward as necessary include the following:

> Radiation Oncologists—Allen Chen, MD, Professor of Radiation Oncology and Vice Chair of Education at the David Geffen School of Medicine at UCLA, says, "Radiation oncologists harness the therapeutic properties of radiation to treat and cure cancer. We are oncologists first, in that we have to understand cancer as a disease, its biology and patterns of spread. Then we determine how radiation fits into the general scheme of treatment."

> Surgical Oncologists—surgical skills are required when a tumor and surrounding tissue need to be removed, when a biopsy is required to help diagnose the cancer, and when reconstruction is indicated in a body area that may have been disfigured or rendered nonfunctional by previous treatment.

> Supportive Care Physicians—doctors who focus on improving a survivor's quality of life by helping manage pain and other symptoms, regardless of whether the cancer is curable, chronic, or life-shortening, regardless of whether the survivor is receiving other treatments, and regardless of whether the survivor is recently diagnosed, in the last stages of life, or anywhere in between.

> Specialists—oncologists who focus on specific cancer types, for example, those treating gynecologic cancers like uterine and cervical, pediatric oncologists treating childhood cancers, and hematologists treating blood cancers.

> Psycho-oncologists—also referred to as psychosocial oncologists— those specializing in helping survivors and families deal with the lifestyle, emotional, behavioral, and social aspects of cancer.

> Pathologists—doctors, typically behind the scenes, who specialize in analyzing cells, tissues, and organs to help with a diagnosis.

> Family Doctors/Primary Care Physicians—although not an oncologist, your family doctor should be expected to coordinate the care for any other medical issues you may have in the context of your cancer.

Supportive Oncology
The Whole Person

Dr. Laura Melton holds a PhD in clinical psychology and is the Medical Director of Supportive Oncology at the University of Colorado Cancer Center. Her organization gives us a view of the kind of support that is available to survivors and their loved ones in coordination with medical oncologists.

Melton is a psycho-oncologist, a mental health provider helping cancer patients cope with and make decisions about their disease, its treatment, and its side effects. She is joined by a cadre of colleagues, all who have special oncology training. They include social workers, registered dieticians, financial counselors, physical and occupational therapists, exercise program leaders, cardiologists, genetic counselors, and fertility specialists.

These disciplines have existed, but until recently, they were not necessarily trained to be oncology-specific, not readily available within cancer centers, and not typically coordinated with the medical oncologists. Recognition that outcomes can be better when care is given to the whole person and not just the disease is fueling the growth of these specially-trained supportive disciplines and organizations.

How you can access this support will vary depending on where you are being treated. Melton's organization is close to, and some are even embedded with, the medical oncologists at the University of Colorado. This model exists at other cancer centers as well. You may, however, be at a cancer center or at a hospital that does not have all of these support disciplines on site. Regardless, you should be asking your doctor or nurse about what support you may need and how to access it.

Because this is a relatively new and growing field of care, even where the support services are integrated into the cancer center, doctors and nurses may not be fully aware of what is available. Melton's Supportive Oncology group is constantly communicating with other medical professionals to ensure they know how she and her colleagues can help.

The support disciplines look to the medical oncologist to be the quarterback of the fully-integrated team. They also make sure that notes of their work with patients are copied to the oncologist and included in the overall medical records.

Melton's team also tends to the needs of a patient's loved ones, conducting support groups, ensuring social workers are being sensitive to caregivers, and even doing research in this area. One such study is assessing the effect on patients receiving bone marrow transplants when the supportive oncology professionals tend to the needs of their caregivers. To date, the more holistic approach is yielding encouraging results.

Melton frequently gets questions from patients about whether they should pursue alternative health approaches versus conventional standards of care. She understands the root of these questions—patients may be fearful of treatments and their side effects and are attracted to what seem like more natural therapies about which they have become aware.

Melton sees her role as helping patients and their loved ones work through these types of critical decisions. She is clear in identifying the risk, similar to that voiced by Dr. John Marshall. If the alternative doesn't work, time has been lost in addressing the cancer, and it may have progressed, making conventional treatment that much more difficult and, perhaps, less likely to succeed.

Other Professionals

During a two-day period in the midst of one of my chemotherapy rounds, I directly interacted with many medical professionals in addition to my oncologist. In this order, I was helped by a phlebotomist who drew my blood for pre-appointment analysis, the nurse practitioner who saw me prior to my visit with Dr. Bartlett, the nurse coordinator, a nurse who conducted my bone marrow biopsy, the clinical trial coordinator, the nurse who inserted an IV for my CT scan, the technician who conducted the CT scan, the primary nurse who saw to my infusions, and the nurses in the infusion pod who verified my medications were correct for quality assurance purposes.

Among those I did not directly see, but who helped, were the laboratory technician who conducted and reported my blood tests, the radiologist who read my CT scan, and the pharmacist who prepared the medications for my infusion.

Each of these medical professionals was an integral member of my support team roster. When I showed up for my appointments and procedures, these experts were present and ready-to-go.

There are other support professionals you may need to identify and recruit to be part of your team, if they are not already coordinated with your medical oncologist.

> ➤ Social worker—survivors and their loved ones frequently need help coping with cancer's challenges. Social workers provide assistance with a wide range of issues from lodging and transportation to rehabilitation and hospice care to advance directives. They also identify resources who can help address issues like legal complications, insurance management, and financial concerns. And they can help directly or suggest options to address coping emotionally. For many survivors, the social worker is the best first contact outside the direct medical oncology team.

> ➤ Physical therapist—functional impairments resulting from cancer symptoms and treatment side effects can sometimes be addressed through physical therapy. Examples of issues a physical therapist can help with are fatigue, pain, balance, and mobility, as well as cardiovascular and neurological impairments. Therapists can also address expected side effects even before treatments begin, sometimes referred to as "pre-habilitation."

> ➤ Occupational therapist—cancer can affect the ability to perform basic activities of daily living. For example, 20% of patients with metastatic disease report cognitive difficulties, and nearly two-thirds report basic functional issues like bending, stooping, lifting, and dressing. The American Occupational Therapy Association, Inc. identifies the role of occupational therapy in oncology as "to facilitate and enable an individual patient to achieve maximum functional performance, both physically and psychologically, in everyday living skills regardless of his or her life expectancy."

> ➤ Genetic counselor—survivors or their relatives may benefit from being tested for gene mutations that have been linked to hereditary risk, such as breast, colon, ovarian, and uterine cancers. Counselors can help determine if genetic testing is appropriate, and if testing is done, they can then help with decisions about prevention or management of cancers, while also providing psychosocial support.

> ➤ Registered dietitian—cancer and its treatment can carry the risk of malnutrition and significant weight loss. Oncology-focused dieticians help patients with nutritional supplements, diet education, feeding tube management, and other services.

Pick Up the Phone

Judy Mange is a physical therapist, certified care manager, former regional manager for the Aging Life Care Association (formerly known as the National Association of Professional Geriatric Care Managers), and the Founder and President of Aging Well, dedicated to helping individuals and families navigate aging, including tending to their health care. Her four-plus decades of experience have enabled her to identify another crucial conversation.

Crucial Conversation Alert

There is always a question of when and when not to call your doctor or seek medical help at the emergency room. We may struggle to balance between our doctors being available to help us manage a health issue yet not wanting to inappropriately call with every little question. Judy Mange counsels that when you have a medical question, it is best to err on the side of caution and go directly to the right source for answers.

She has observed that at times, her clients are hesitant to call their doctor when, in her judgement, a call could have prevented some issues. There may be any number of reasons for this. They may "not want to bother the doctor" with something that may not be serious. They may not want to hear bad news that may derive from the call. They may be in denial that there is anything wrong. They may be concerned about the costs of what might ensue. They don't have "the time to be sick." They may not want to burden loved ones with "yet another" trip to the doctor or emergency room.

When is the right time to contact your doctor? If it is the right time, will you do so? How will you make contact? If the answers to these questions are not clear, it's time for a crucial conversation with your doctor.

When I had my first appointment with Dr. Bartlett to monitor my CLL progression, she provided me a three-ring binder with general information about cancer. It also contains tabs in which I can collect additional information about treatment, resources, and survivorship. The first page is in a clear plastic protective sleeve and is much more specific. It contains the names and phone numbers of the people in Dr. Bartlett's office that I might need to contact and a very detailed explanation of when it is right to call.

There are 15 listed conditions that include things like a temperature over 100, a persistent cough, weakness or dizziness, and skin rash. I've called several times over the years and talked to Nurse Coordinator Susan Young, RN. She's done a great job of understanding the reason for my call and guiding me to the right indicated action or to a decision that no action is needed.

That being said, I find it difficult to determine when it's appropriate to make the call. Over time, I've opted to be on the safe side and pick up the phone.

In Chapter 8, you'll be building your medical and supportive oncology team. Doing so will build confidence, which will further build hope.

Take a moment to capture your thoughts for this chapter.

1. What are the three key ideas I learned from this chapter?
2. Based on what I learned in this chapter:
   a. What will I want to build into my plans?
   b. Who might help me do this?

Chapter 5

How Can We Help?
Support Community

---

*"To the world you may be one person;
but to one person you may be the world."*
Dr. Seuss

"So that no one faces cancer alone."
Cancer Support Community

Doing Good

Pillowcases:

A woman walks into the infusion pod carrying a box. She comes up to my chair first, eventually visiting each of us, and says, "Have you gotten a pillowcase?"

I shake my head, and she continues, "I'd like you to have one. I've been in your chair, and my friends brought me quilts they made to keep me warm during my treatments. I knew I couldn't do that for everyone, so I make pillowcases."

I asked her how she was doing, and she said, "I'm two-and-a-half years since my pancreatic cancer diagnosis, and I'm doing well."

I thank her for the pillowcase and tell her, "You're doing well by doing good."

Thanksgiving:

A woman walks into the pod the day before Thanksgiving. She has several nurses in tow, and leads her contingent around the pod collecting other nurses and hospital staff. When her group is assembled, she declares so that everyone can hear, "I came by to thank you for keeping me alive this year. I have a lot to be thankful for, including all of you." Then she distributed warm home-baked cookies.

Therapy Dogs:

Two women enter the pod, each with a well-behaved dog on a leash. They circulate, asking patients if they would like a "therapy dog" visit. Most say yes, giving license to the dogs, each trained for this service, to make themselves available to be petted and hugged.

These animals and their human partners can make a noticeable difference in the emotional wellbeing of cancer patients. One of the dog's handlers explains that therapy dog programs exist at some, and a growing number, of cancer treatment centers. The program at my St. Louis Siteman Cancer Center is lovingly called TOUCH, Therapy of Unique Canine Helpers.

As these examples just begin to demonstrate, there is support all around us, sometimes where you least expect it. There are individuals and networks and organizations. Your opportunity is to be open to listening and looking for the support you might need and then decide what you believe will really help you. Sometimes it just shows up—sometimes you have to seek it out. For me, a pillowcase and hearing others be thankful, cookies included—yes, thank you. Therapy dog—no, thank you.

Although the support community for cancer survivors and caregivers is too extensive to fully describe, throughout the remainder of this chapter we'll look at other examples to get a broader sense of what is available and how to access it.

It's All for the Kids

In 1987, Allen Brockman was volunteering at Children's Hospital in St. Louis and was moved in two ways. He was moved emotionally, as he connected with the kids who had cancer and other serious diseases. And he was moved to act.

Allen and his wife, Ronnie, took a leap of faith to found what would be called Camp Rainbow, a sleepaway experience for children with cancer. Over the 30-plus ensuing years, they created four additional camping experiences: a day camp for kids with cancer, ages four to six, Teen Camp for high schoolers, Family Camp, and the Camp-In program for which the camp comes to the hospitals to create an experience for those who are unable to make it to remote locations.

At the sleepaway camp for ages six to thirteen, each day is themed and includes a morning full of activities, an afternoon activity led by local volunteer crafts people, an afternoon rest period, sno-cones every day, three great meals, and an evening activity. Sound like a normal camp? That's because it is. Yes, the campers have cancer. Yes, there is a counselor for each camper. Yes, the camp is situated within minutes of a hospital. Yes, the camp has medical staff and facilities that go well beyond most sleepaway camps. Oh, and yes, it's free to everyone.

But to the kids and their parents, Camp Rainbow is a respite from the effects of cancer and its treatment. It is a week full of fun, of making and building friendships, of creating positive memories.

Campers are selected by three local hospitals. First-time parents are more than hesitant about sending their child away for a week; a child who may not have been out of their sight since diagnosis. These concerns are allayed by the hospital staff, camp leadership, and experienced parents, all who reach out to help new parents envision the week.

By day two, the parents, who have dropped their kids off and gotten a few final questions answered before leaving, are relaxed, with the camp staff in phone contact as needed. By the end of the week, the parents are already lobbying for their child to return to camp the following year and offering to volunteer in any capacity for which they may be needed.

Not only is the camp wonderful for their kids, it is a respite for the parents to find time for each other and for their other children. Everybody wins, but as the Brockmans say, "It's all for the kids."

One of the byproducts of the Camp Rainbow experience is the creation of an extended family of families that acts as an engaged and active support system. Many of the families knew each other previously through their common experience and shared time at the local hospitals. But the camp brings kids, parents, and staff together in a new, more intimate way. Unfortunately, this plays out all-too-frequently when a camper passes away, and the Camp Rainbow community rallies around to offer support.

One of the measures of Camp Rainbow's success is that many of the counselors and both medical and non-medical staff are former campers who want to give back to others by creating the experience they so fondly remember.

And why not? Those who don't know Camp Rainbow might well think it is a depressing place with all of the young cancer survivors. Yet, as Ronnie Brockman says that not unlike other oncology camps (there is an international organization called the Children's Oncology Camping Association, made up of over 125 independent camps that serve more than 42,000 kids with cancer every year) and camps for other childhood diseases, "It's the happiest place in the world."

Good for a Lifetime

Camp Rainbow gives every camper a knotted rawhide ring about an inch in diameter. The ring holds three silvery metal tokens, each about the size of a quarter. Each token has a figure cutout in the middle through which the rawhide is strung.

One token cutout is a dove—on one side is etched "faith token" and on the other side "believe in miracles."

A second token's cutout is a moon and star—on one side is "dream token" and on the other "reach for the stars."

The third token's cutout is a butterfly—"friendship token" and "good for a lifetime."

The Brockmans report that it is not uncommon for campers who return as staff or who they see many years later still have their ring of tokens, many who carry it with them always.

In 1995, Nicole Giamanco was diagnosed with a rare form of leukemia, enduring extensive hospital stays, frequently in intensive care, and more than two years of chemotherapy. A bright light for her was Camp Rainbow.

Although Giamanco wanted to be a doctor even before she was diagnosed, her experience with the medical professionals who cared for her helped her choose her specialty. Nicole Giamanco, MD is a Pediatric Hematologist-Oncologist in Tacoma, Washington, where she also teaches medical school students when they are on rotations.

And she still has her Camp Rainbow rawhide token ring—"good for a lifetime."

On a personal note—after the Brockmans and I finished discussing their section of the book, they were kind enough to present me with a Camp Rainbow rawhide token ring. I immediately put it on my keychain. When they gave it to me, they were unaware of my CLL diagnosis, but I feel additionally protected by the friendship with which they gave it. Yes, "good for a lifetime."

Pay It Forward

Although Rick Hitt is retired from a successful career in the advertising/public relations/communications business, he continually looks for ways to "keep the juices flowing" by applying his skills and experiences to help others. The Lumina program at Barnes-Jewish-Christian (BJC) Health Systems in St. Louis has enabled Hitt to do just that.

Lumina offers hospice care patients of all ages a variety of ways to capture their legacy, and then provides trained volunteers to make it happen. Survivors and their families can choose to develop such options as scrapbooks, memory books, family trees, and a letter to loved ones.

Hitt, who has a journalism degree, loves writing and storytelling. He applies this expertise and passion to interview the patient and their family members, and he reviews other information provided by the family. For example, he was able to glean insights about one patient's life from greeting cards sent by friends and relatives. Hitt then combined visuals and text to tell the patient's story. The result was a professionally printed and bound legacy book.

Through BJC's generosity and Hitt's volunteered dedication of time and talent, the Lumina program is free to families. Although the patients and their families greatly appreciate what he does for them, Hitt benefits as well as he is allowed the opportunity "to pay it forward."

Sense of Comfort

The Brockmans, Rick Hitt, the pillowcase maker, the Thanksgiving survivor, and the therapy dog handlers are but a few who are examples of the many who support survivors and their loved ones. Two others are Sister Carla Mae Streeter of the Dominican Order and Rabbi Jeffrey Stiffman.

Rabbi Stiffman was ordained in 1965 at the Hebrew Union College-Jewish Institute of Religion, and he earned his PhD in Theology in 1972. He retired as the Senior Rabbi of Congregation Shaare Emeth in St. Louis in 2004 and has continued to serve as Rabbi Emeritus.

One of the many roles he has filled over his greater than five decades in the rabbinate is that of pastoral counselor for the ill, including cancer survivors, and their families. It is a role that he refers to as one of being a "caring listener" to provide a "sense of comfort."

Stiffman has helped those who believed in God and those who did not; those who believed that God would get them through the ordeal and those who lost faith in a God who would put them through it; those who wanted to pray; those who wanted to hold his hand; those who wanted his advice about faith and those who wanted advice about cancer; those who wanted to just sit quietly and those who wanted a caring listener with whom to share their feelings; those who had given up and those who revealed an inner strength. There were those he visited in hospitals, those he visited at home, and those who joined him for healing services.

Because every patient and family member is different, Stiffman sees his role of pastoral counselor as one of profoundly understanding the needs and desires of the individual, then either personally helping or suggesting other resources. He is a believer in support groups, whether they be faith-based or not, that can provide an additional place to talk through issues, especially for those who may have little or no local family or friend support.

Sister Carla Mae Streeter is a Dominican sister, Doctor of Theology, and Professor Emerita of Systematic Theology and Spirituality at Aquinas Institute of Theology. She formerly served on the Board of the Interfaith Partnership of Metropolitan St. Louis and presently serves on the Board of the Institute for the Theological Encounter with Science and Technology. She is the first woman to complete a theological doctorate at Regis University in Toronto.

Streeter suggests that the sadness, fear, anger, and other emotions the survivor and loved ones are experiencing can only be dealt with when brought to the surface. She views her role of mentor for the ill as walking beside them hand-in-hand, both figuratively and literally. In doing so, she helps them formulate the questions by which they learn more about their circumstances and themselves, helps them acknowledge their reality, helps them make medical and personal decisions, and helps them take the appropriate actions—all things that may be difficult to do without caring, and perhaps spiritual, support.

Recall that our model for building hope includes building confidence and part of doing so is exploring your spirituality, whether your belief system is rooted in organized religion or you approach this aspect of life in a private way. Clergy like Rabbi Stiffman and Sister Streeter may be a resource to help you do just that.

The late Debbie Friedman was a musician, singer, and songwriter of Jewish melodies with a passion for helping people heal physically, emotionally, and spiritually. She wrote a prayer for healing that is used widely in synagogues, homes, hospitals, and wherever and whenever its message is needed. Among its lyrics:

> *Bless those in need of healing with r'fuah sh'leimah,*
>> (Hebrew transliteration meaning "complete healing")
> *The renewal of body, the renewal of spirit,*
> *And let us say, Amen*

Caregiving—It's about the Survivor

The cancer community is full of those who are available to support survivors. Many just show up and others need to be sought out. As a survivor, you can be mindful about who you want on your team by assessing the relative benefits of each possible supporter.

You may not want a pillowcase, regardless of how well-intentioned the craftsperson might be. You may not want a visit from a therapy dog. You may choose not to spend time with a pastoral counselor. But there is one support-team member virtually no one opts out of—a loved one, either a family member or friend, who takes the lead role of primary caregiver.

It is an understatement that this support role is critical to the survivor, and it is a role that so many of us have played, are playing, or will play. Recall that about 40% of us will be diagnosed with cancer in our lifetime. One could argue that means that at least 40% of us will be a caregiver for a survivor in our lifetime.

Former First Lady Rosalynn Carter once said, "There are only four kinds of people in this world—those who have been caregivers, those who are currently caregivers, those who will be caregivers, and those who need caregivers."

For the sake of this discussion, we'll talk about the primary caregiver as one individual, although it can be a small group, like siblings sharing the responsibility for a parent or a couple supporting a child.

Also for our purposes, we'll use the word caregiver to mean what many refer to as an "informal caregiver," which is distinguished from a "formal caregiver," one who does the work professionally and is, therefore, paid for the services.

Crucial Conversation Alert

Whether you have previously been on either side of the patient/ caregiver relationship or whether this is your first time, it is of value to have the crucial conversations to make sure you are aligned to each other's expectations. Here are a number of topics worth discussing and some suggestions about what the expectations might be:

➤ Although there may be times when the caregiver may feel the need to step in to make decisions or take charge, the preference is to defer to the survivor if he or she has the wherewithal. If for example, the caregiver has a different point of view from the survivor about the best course of treatment, it is right to clearly share that point of view but then leave the final decision up to the survivor—again, assuming he or she has the wherewithal to do so. Remember, it's about the survivor. There are times when the caregiver does, in fact, need to take charge, for example, if you are the parent of a child survivor or a child of an elderly parent who can no longer make decisions on his or her own.

➤ The survivor should be the primary communicator with doctors. The loved one may help by listening and taking notes about what is said or by formulating questions before appointments. But during the sessions, unless the survivor asks for help, the caregiver's role is one of active listener.

> ➤ Organizing all of the paperwork such as test results, insurance forms, treatment records, contact information, and appointment schedules can be an onerous task. It's helpful to figure out who will do what to make sure there's no duplication and nothing falls through the cracks.

> ➤ As a loved one, you can be a major source of inspiration in many circumstances, perhaps for example, encouraging the survivor to adhere to a demanding treatment plan. As with all of these topics, it will have been helpful to have had a crucial conversation before the need arises.

> ➤ The caregiver and survivor should agree on the what, when, and how to keep other family members and friends informed—the loved one may need to be the outward communicator.

> ➤ The caregiver and survivor should agree on what practical help the caregiver will provide or will make arrangements with other resources to deliver. As but a few examples, who will do the grocery shopping and manage meals, provide transportation, help around the house, tend to financial matters?

Caregiver—Take Good Care of You

As a loved one, you can be the foundation of the survivor's support system, but you may need support as well. Recall how Camp Rainbow provided not only a meaningful experience for the kids, but it also provided a much-needed respite for parents and siblings.

Your loved one's cancer diagnosis and all that comes with it profoundly affects you as well. If you're like most loved ones in a caregiver role, you'll find yourself intimately sharing the survivor's emotional rollercoaster while also experiencing your own ups and downs. Some would refer to you as a "co-survivor."

Loved ones both provide and need support. You have your own fears and worries. You are under stress as well. Your energy may be drained. Your schedule may become challenging. Your work and your finances may be affected.

In their document, *Caring for the Caregiver*, the National Cancer Institute says it well, "While giving care, it's normal to put your own needs and feelings aside. But putting your needs aside for a long time is not good for your health. You need to take care of yourself, too. If you don't, you may not be able to care for others. This is why you need to take good care of you."

In her book, *Choose Hope (Always Choose Hope)*, Elizabeth Clark emphasizes this concept with a single powerful word, "burnout." She writes, "Burnout is a state of emotional exhaustion," and adds, "Living with uncertainty and setbacks is exhausting. Families under stress have a decreased ability to make decisions or solve problems. They recognize that moving forward is important, but they may not know how to do so."

You can benefit by being open to asking for help, which is sometimes a hard thing to do. You may join a support group, where you can talk with other caregivers about your feelings and seek advice. You will want to be sensitive to monitoring your own health—as difficult as it may seem, discipline yourself to get sufficient rest, take mindful steps to reduce stress, eat healthily, exercise, and if you are on your own medication regimen, adhere to it.

Perhaps the best way to care for yourself is to make sure you attend to building hope, to be clear about developing both your cancer and non-cancer life plans, and to build your own support team. Yes, it's important that you help your loved-one survivor to do these things, but not to the exclusion of you doing them as well. It's also about you.

Caregiving—Other Factors

As you strive to do what's best for the survivor and for yourself, there are a number of other possible factors regarding caregiving that would be worth your consideration at the appropriate time.

> ➤ Planning is likely to be more complex and the situation more financially challenging if you live far from the survivor you are supporting. It may be that you live across town in a large city whereby quick trips to the survivor are not possible, or you may live out of town. Not only should the cancer plan include day-to-day care/support details to account for the distance, but it should also include an answer to the question, "What happens if there is an emergency and I can't get there quickly?"

> ➤ Proximity may not be the only location concern. You may live close to the survivor, but you are in a rural community with more difficult access to physicians and treatment services. This situation may affect transportation, finances, and fundamentally, the quality of care.

> ➤ Even a brief respite from caregiving has benefits, whether it is sending your child to an experience like Camp Rainbow to provide you a week to focus on other people and things, or finding a way to take a daily walk to both get exercise and relieve some stress, or planning to share caregiving time with other family and friends. Mindfully building respite care into your plan is an important aspect of protecting your own physical and mental wellbeing.

> ➤ Caregiving can carry significant financial consequences, especially in a long-term situation. If the caregiver role affects your ability to work, you may forego wages, possibly affecting Social Security and pension benefits. About two-thirds of family caregivers report conflicts between their jobs and their caregiving role, sometimes needing to take unpaid leave and/or a reduction in work hours. This issue sits on top of a possible loss of income for the survivor, if he or she has also needed to reduce work hours or even leave the job, perhaps putting employer-based medical benefits at risk.

> ➤ There may be legal considerations as well. If the survivor may become unable to make health care and financial decisions, if you haven't already, make sure you put the right documents in place to enable you to legally make decisions in their stead. Documents may include a general durable power of attorney and a durable power of attorney for health care.

One common theme that runs through all of the considerations of caregiving is that, just like the patient, you will benefit from thoughtful planning versus waiting for issues to arise and dealing with them reactively. When we get to Chapters 8 and 9, develop your own cancer and non-cancer plans, including establishing your support team. As caregiver, developing your plans and team is in your best interest and thereby in the best interest of the patient.

And to reemphasize, each of these considerations, if they apply to you, is typically better to address sooner rather than later.

Run the Experiment

Whether you are a survivor or a loved one, live alone or are surrounded by family and friends, are an extrovert or introvert, it is worthwhile to consider what organized support communities and support groups can do for you.

One of the many organizations that facilitates such groups and provides survivors and loved ones with other support opportunities has the appropriate name of the Cancer Support Community. It is international in scope with locations in 22 states, the District of Columbia, as well as Canada, Israel, and Japan.

Its history goes back to 1982, when Harriett and Dr. Harold Benjamin founded The Wellness Community in Santa Monica, California. They were inspired to do so by Harriett's breast cancer diagnosis in 1972. Although she responded well to treatment, eventually living more than 35 years cancer-free, the Benjamins recognized the unmet need of supporting survivors and their loved ones socially and emotionally. The Wellness Community offered 25 support groups per week at no cost.

The approach gained momentum thanks to Gilda Radner, an original cast member on *Saturday Night Live*, who was diagnosed with stage IV ovarian cancer in 1986. Radner discovered The Wellness Community, mentioned the organization in her book, *It's Always Something*, and wrote of what she learned there, "The goal is to have a full, productive life, even with all that ambiguity. No matter what happens, whether the cancer never flares up again, or whether you die, the important thing is that the days you have had, you will have LIVED...I've learned that what I can control is whether I am going to live a day in fear and depression and panic, or whether I am going to attack the day and make it as good a day, as wonderful a day, as I can."

After Radner died in 1989, her husband, comedic actor Gene Wilder, and others began a Wellness Community-like organization on the East Coast they called Gilda's Club. Each of the organizations expanded to other cities over the years and in 2009, chose to merge into the Cancer Support

Community. Its mission remains fully consistent with the vision the Benjamins had decades before, "to ensure that all people impacted by cancer are empowered by knowledge, strengthened by action, and sustained by community to enhance their overall wellbeing." And, it's still all at no cost.

Renata Sledge, MSW, LCSW is Program Director at the Cancer Support Community of Greater St. Louis and is responsible for organizing and facilitating many of the activities that address each of the three tenets of the mission.

"Empowered by Knowledge" programs cover a wide range of relevant education topics. Just a few examples are how to communicate about your cancer, the role genetics plays, and how to approach intimacy and sexual wellness.

"Strengthened by Action" programs speak to healthy lifestyle and stress management. Examples include mindful eating, creative journaling, and restorative movement to improve balance, strength, and bone health.

"Sustained by Community" programs have a social focus. Examples include crafts groups, discussions about hope, and community meals.

At the core of the programming are the support and networking groups. These professionally-facilitated groups are conducted in comfortable, welcoming spaces, frequently in partnership with other community cancer organizations. The groups bring together those with similar diagnoses or life circumstances to meaningfully connect with and learn from each other.

On but one given day of the Cancer Support Community calendar are Tai Chi, Open Art Studio, Energy 101: Balancing Your Body's Energy, Gynecological Cancer Networking Group, and Survivorship Series Networking Group. On another day is Yoga, Line Dancing, Monthly Men's Breakfast, Breast Cancer Networking Group, and Family, Food, and Fun. And another is Zumba, Family and Friends Support Group, Bereavement Support Group, and Mindful Practice.

You may be asking yourself whether a community approach like this is right for you. It is a personal decision based on whether you believe you would benefit. Are you outgoing or a more private person? Do you have sufficient information to manage your cancer experience or might you learn from others? Do you feel you have others on your current support team that you can share with or do you think you would benefit from talking with others who are sharing similar experiences?

Sledge suggests that perhaps the best way to help you answer these questions is try a group or activity at your local support organization. You may want to run the experiment.

Stupid Cancer

The Stupid Cancer home page starts out, "welcome to the club you didn't ask to join. we know you're pissed. and that's OK. we've been there, too. we connect you with your community and strive to make it all suck a little less."

This is not likely the language of a newly diagnosed 72-year-old grandmother or a nine-year-old survivor. It is the language of its target audience, the approximately 72,000 young adults, ages 15 to 39, who are diagnosed in the U.S. every year. This cancer cohort is unique in several ways: 1) survival rates are not increasing as successfully as those for older adults or children; 2) health issues may be different, like dealing with risks of infertility at a time of life when that is most important; and 3) they may be living on their own for the first time adding to the risk of isolation, may be in a new marriage and building a family, or may be in the very heart of establishing a career.

Stupid Cancer exists "to ensure that no one affected by young adult cancer go unaware of the age-appropriate support resources they need so that they can get busy living."

To get a sense of their support connections, one need only click on one of the subjects in Stupid Cancer's "what can we make suck less?" section: "i'm all alone," "i need money," "insurance sucks," "i need a lawyer," i can't work," "am i fertile?" Or you can join other young-adult survivors and caregivers at Stupid Cancer's annual CancerCon, nearly four days of networking with peers who "get it," of education sessions, and of just plain fun.

Robert Roesler de Villers

On October 20, 1944, 16-year old Robert Roesler de Villers died of leukemia. After five years of mourning, Robbie's parents, Rudolph and Antoinette, began a fundraising and education organization in his name.

At the time, leukemia was "...100% fatal...almost a unique situation among the many diseases to which man is susceptible." The de Villers foundation continued to grow and to focus on finding cures for all blood cancers and on improving the quality of life of patients and their families.

Although the name changed over the years to eventually become the Leukemia & Lymphoma Society, the mission has remained the same, and now LLS is the world's largest voluntary health organization dedicated to funding blood cancer research.

LLS is also another example of a cancer organization that offers support services and education for survivors and caregivers. Search cancer organizations and find one that most closely matches your diagnosis and needs. The LLS website, for example, leads you to the following support services:

> ➤ Information Specialists: a staff of "master's level oncology social workers, nurses, and health educators" who are available via phone, chat, and email to help with up-to-date information about treatment and available support
> ➤ Peer-to-Peer Support: a program that connects recently diagnosed blood cancer survivors or their loved ones with trained peer volunteers who have gone through a similar experience
> ➤ Clinical Trial Specialists: a staff that can help you find an appropriate clinical trial and guide you through the clinical-trial process
> ➤ Financial Assistance: qualified patients have access to an insurance "Co-Pay Assistance Program" and a "Patient Travel Assistance Program," as well as access to guidance and tools to navigate the complexity of health insurance and claims filing
> ➤ Family Support Groups: local LLS chapters conduct free support groups, facilitated by credentialed health professionals, where families can learn from each other and share feelings in a comfortable and caring environment
> ➤ Weekly Online Chat for Caregivers: this is moderated by an oncology social worker and is but one of many caregiver support offerings

By the way, since the time of Robbie's death, when leukemia was "100% fatal," leukemia survival has continued to improve. In the early 1960's, the five-year survival rate was 14%. This increased to 34% by the mid-1970's and to 63% in the time frame of 2006 to 2012.

Take a moment to capture your thoughts for this chapter.

1. What are the three key ideas I learned from this chapter?
2. Based on what I learned in this chapter:
   a. What will I want to build into my plans?
   b. Who might help me do this?

Chapter 6

We're Working on It
Researchers

"Medical science has proven time and again
that when the resources are provided,
great progress in the treatment, cure,
and prevention of disease can occur."
Michael J. Fox

"I pictured myself as a virus or a cancer cell
and tried to sense what it would be like..."
Jonas Salk

Nonstop Work

When I was working at the Procter & Gamble Company, a colleague left the company to fulfill her dream of owning and growing her own business. After developing an A-list of possible ventures and doing a lot of research, she purchased a horse trailer manufacturing business. Twenty-five years later, she sold the business at an attractive price and retired. When I congratulated her on the sale, she smiled wryly and replied, "It only took me 25 years of nonstop work to become an overnight success."

Her statement also serves to describe the cancer research community, its work, its timelines, and its successes. When your oncologist recommends a given treatment for your particular cancer, its availability has been preceded by decades of creativity, science, organization, dedication, setbacks, funding, approvals, and other predictable and unpredictable parts of the process. It has been preceded by the nonstop work of researchers and the trust and hope of clinical trial participants, people like you and me.

Along the way, researchers have been educated and trained. Facilities have been built and equipped. Ideas have germinated and been tested at the lab bench. Animal testing and human clinical trials have been conducted. Academics have collaborated across the country and around the world. Priority decisions have been made on which of the many diseases to work on and which studies to pursue. Pharmaceutical companies have chosen to participate and to build manufacturing and marketing capability. The Food and Drug Administration (FDA) has become involved and, when appropriate, provided their approval. Patents have been filed. Physicians across cancer centers have been educated on the new approach. Researchers have studied how the new approach will work across population demographics and have sought to find ways to ensure access to the improved treatment across those demographics. And for all of this, funding has been developed and allocated.

So we sit in the oncologist's office, generally unaware of what has gone into making our treatment available and into creating part of our foundation for hope. To paraphrase my former colleague, "It took the cancer community many years of nonstop work to create an overnight success."

In this chapter, we'll learn more about cancer research. Can we find reasons to critique the cancer research community? Yes. Is the treatment development process long and expensive? Yes. Is the cost of the resultant therapies high? Frequently. But has the community made progress, and does it continue to do so? Absolutely.

AML Master Trial

Amy Burd, PhD, is Vice President of Research Strategy at the Leukemia & Lymphoma Society and former Oncology Portfolio Manager at Bayer Pharmaceuticals. In her spare time, she is a biotechnology consultant.

As if all of that weren't enough, Burd also spends what she describes as 120% of her time as the leader of a complex and critical multi-organizational research team to conduct the "Beat AML Master Trial." AML (acute myeloid leukemia) is a blood cancer that is responsible for over 10,000 deaths per year in the U.S. alone.

The trial's objective is to change how AML is treated by finding the specific genetic mutations that cause the disease and developing the drug or drug combination that will precisely address each particular mutation.

Burd's leadership brings together a collaboration among LLS, many prominent academic cancer centers, and a number of biopharmaceutical firms.

Understanding how the Beat AML Master Trial came to be, its timeline, and how it will play out in the future is a great example of how the research community works and will work.

LLS, like all cancer research funding institutions, manages a delicate balance to ensure their financial and human resources are best used. They constantly monitor where the needs are greatest (the standard of care for AML has not changed in 40 years, and the five-year survival rate has seen little improvement relative to other cancers—remaining below 20% for patients over 60) and where the research seems to be heading (the learning has been emerging that AML is not a single disease but rather a multitude of diseases, each with a different genomic mutation). LLS was already spending a quarter of its research budget on AML and more grant applications were coming in all of the time. They asked, "What if the work could be coordinated across all researchers working in the AML space?"

Burd started with a group of nearly 20 thought leaders, then over time grew the group to more than 100 people to include more researchers, the FDA, and nearly 30 interested pharmaceutical companies. The FDA's close involvement facilitated approval of the trial's protocol, and the Beat AML Master Trial was launched.

The trial has ten study arms, each applying a different drug regimen to a specific genomic mutation. It will eventually be conducted across 15 to 20 cancer centers in order to accrue sufficient trial participants to meet the goal of 500 over the five years of the study. And there will be five or more pharmaceutical firms participating, adding to the impressive and perhaps unprecedented collaboration.

Along the way, the need for another breakthrough has been identified and its solution is being developed. The process to analyze a patient's genomics and diagnose the disease currently takes two to three weeks. AML is an aggressive cancer, and any time saved in diagnosis is critical. The study is requiring only a seven-day turnaround of genomic testing and diagnosis to optimize patient survival rates, and the team is figuring out how to meet that need.

At the end of the trial, it is expected that the study will have demonstrated which drug regimen can become the new AML standard of care for each of its genomic mutations. Those drugs will then be translated into manufactured products by the pharmaceutical companies with the approval of the FDA, which continues to stay close to the trial.

When that happens, the time from that first thought-leader meeting called by LLS to the availability of an improved standard of care for AML patients will have been many years, not even counting the decades of basic research that took place before the initial group got together to envision the Beat AML Master Trial.

Clinical Trial Participation

An issue that the Beat AML Master Trial faces is one confronted by every clinical trial, regardless of its size and complexity—ensuring there are sufficient participants. The cancer research community calls it "accrual." You can make a more informed decision about your own participation in a trial if you know more about what they are and know what to ask your doctor.

Clinical trials are conducted in phases, with each phase having a specific objective. On its way to approval, a new drug or new therapy is required to go through each of three phases and maybe a fourth.

Phase I: This phase answers two questions, "What is the right dosage?" and "Is the treatment safe?" Typically, a few people get a small dose and are then monitored for side effects. If side effects are minor, dosages are increased for the next small group of participants. Close monitoring continues. In this way, a safe level of the drug is determined.

Phase II: This phase answers the question, "Does the treatment work?" An increased number of patients, as many as 100, with the similar type of cancer get the same drug. Both the benefits and side effects of the treatment are closely monitored. If there are meaningful benefits without major side effects, the drug can go on to Phase III.

Phase III: This phase answers the question, "Is it better than what's already available?" Both safety and effectiveness of the new treatment are compared against the current standard of care. To insure the integrity of the trial, participants are randomly assigned which treatment they will get, either the trial therapy or the current standard. The number of participants increases over Phases I and II, with several hundred usually needed to answer the research question. As with previous phases, patients are closely monitored. If new unacceptable side effects are detected, a decision may be made to stop the study. Some eligible trial candidates are concerned about being assigned to a part of the study that uses a placebo, a substance with no therapeutic effect. Placebos are never used in Phase I and II studies. They may be used at Phase III, but not if there's a current standard treatment available that works, and you would be informed of this when you consent to participate in the study. An example of how placebos might be used is to assess whether adding a new drug to the standard of care works better—in this case, the two arms of the study might be standard of care plus placebo versus standard of care plus the new drug.

Phase IV: When a Phase III trial is successful as measured by improved effectiveness and/or safety, a New Drug Application (NDA) is submitted to the FDA for approval. If the FDA approves the new treatment, it becomes a new standard of care. The FDA can also choose to approve the NDA but ask that the new treatment be formally monitored over time to gain additional data on a larger sampling. Phase IV answers the question, "What else do we need to know?" Monitoring may take place on thousands of patients over many years.

At each phase of the research, a trial goes through many scientific reviews and approvals before participants are exposed. The effect of the trial on patients is of utmost concern with the intent that neither effectiveness of treatment nor safety is compromised.

For example, I participated in a Phase III clinical trial when it was time for treatment for my CLL. I was randomly assigned to the arm of the trial in which the current standard of care would be administered. The study then included an assessment as to whether my treatment was working. If it were not, the design of the study was such that I would have immediately been switched to the trial drug, although not all studies are designed with a "crossover" treatment option. It was clear to me when I agreed to be on the study that my wellbeing would not be sacrificed for the sake of gathering data.

Did you know?

➤ At any given time, there may be as many as 800 new anticancer drugs in various stages of development.

➤ About 3% of adult cancer patients participate in a clinical trial.

➤ 40% of trials for adults fail to achieve their minimum accrual targets.

➤ For phase III trials for adults, more than 60% do not reach minimum accrual.

➤ More than 60% of children being treated for cancer are part of a clinical trial.

Your Trial Participation

Crucial Conversation Alert

One of the questions we identified in Chapter 2 that you may want to ask your doctor is, "How can I learn about and access clinical trials that apply to me?"

You can also find a wealth of information about current clinical trial options at cancer.gov, the website of the National Cancer Institute at the National Institutes of Health. Go to "About Cancer" – then "Treatment" – then "Clinical Trials" – then "Find NCI-Supported Clinical Trials." You may also find clinical trial information about your specific cancer at relevant web sites. For example, Fight Colorectal Cancer has a Clinical Trial Finder.

Were you to participate in a clinical trial, you would be in as direct contact with the cancer research community as you would likely ever be. But why should you or should you not be in a trial? The subject of participating in a clinical trial is a discussion to have with your doctor and with other resources who can help you understand the benefits and risks. You'll not be enrolled in a trial until you review and sign a consent document agreeing to participate. It is your right to withdraw from a trial at any time.

Your reasons to be on a trial may be altruistic, personal, or both. You may want to be a part of creating a better future for others who share your cancer or who have yet to be diagnosed. Clinical trials serve to advance science, and you may choose to be a part of something larger than yourself.

It is also perfectly acceptable to be selfish about joining a trial. Your doctor and you can assess the odds that the current standard of care will work for you. If you are concerned about that or if you've already received the standard of care and it was not successful, your oncologist can help you understand the potential effects of the trial treatment.

Regardless of what you eventually choose to do, make sure you base your decision on all of the relevant information. The National Coalition for Cancer Survivorship recommends you ask and understand the answers to these questions:

- ➢ Why would this trial be important to me? What is the aim of the study?
- ➢ What are the potential risks and benefits to me compared to other treatment options I have?
- ➢ What are the eligibility requirements?
- ➢ Who will monitor my care and safety?
- ➢ What are the trial's tests and treatments? Will I need to be in the hospital, and if so, how often and for how long?
- ➢ How do the possible side effects of the study treatment compare to the side effects of the standard treatment option?
- ➢ What support will be there for me and my caregivers during the trial? Can I talk to someone if I have questions?
- ➢ Will my insurance, Medicaid, Medicare, or managed care plan cover costs of the trial? Who will help me answer these coverage questions?
- ➢ What are my responsibilities and out-of-pocket costs?
- ➢ What is the long-term follow-up care?

Just as the choice of standard treatment options is yours, so is the choice whether or not to participate in a clinical trial.

The Whole Person

Cathy Bradley, PhD, is Associate Director of Cancer Prevention and Control at the University of Colorado Cancer Center and was previously the founding Chair of the Department of Healthcare Policy and Research at Virginia Commonwealth University School of Medicine. Her current role opens our window on another aspect of the cancer research community, that of population research.

Population research occurs outside the controlled environments of the laboratory and clinical trials, which, Bradley points out, are critical to fundamental understanding and the demonstration of effectiveness and safety, but they have their limitations.

This research approach studies the general population as well as subsets of interest. Studies are conducted on such topics as broad health outcomes, the economic impact of disease on individuals and society at large, and effects on employment, a particular focus of Dr. Bradley's. In recent years, there has been a trend to study caregivers as well as survivors, the hypothesis being that if caregivers are healthier, so will be survivors.

The results of population research can serve to inform individual patients to enable better treatment decision making and can serve to inform cancer institutions and policy makers with regards to the effects of cancer on public health.

A clinical trial may demonstrate, for example, that a new drug reduces the size of tumors but identifies that some patients experience peripheral neuropathy, numbness, weakness, and pain in hands and feet. Population research following this clinical trial might then study the effects of the therapy on the whole person, perhaps finding survivors are having a difficult time returning to work because of the neuropathy. The results of such a study could then be shared by doctors so that patients can make more fully-informed treatment decisions.

Perhaps the foremost example of how population research can affect public policy is the studies that demonstrated the serious effects of smoking on cancer incidence and mortality. The American Association for Cancer

Research estimates that "more than 8 million smoking-related deaths were prevented from 1964 to 2014 because of declines in cigarette smoking rates."

Another example comes from Bradley's own work, which frequently focuses on underserved and minority populations. Her paper published in the *Journal of the National Cancer Institute* reported findings that regardless of socioeconomic status, African-American women are diagnosed later and die more often from breast cancer than white women.

Having the data can lead to the appropriate actions.

Animal Oncology

Carrissa Wood, DVM, is a Doctor of Veterinary Medicine at IndyVet and formerly a Veterinary Medical Oncology Resident Instructor with the department of Small Animal Oncology at the Texas A&M University Veterinary Medical Teaching Hospital. She is working in the growing field of animal oncology, both seeing patients and instructing other veterinarians.

Wait! What? Why should we pay attention to cancer in our pets? Two reasons—people care about their pets, and the development of animal oncology is enhancing both diagnostic and therapeutic capability for people.

Depending on the source of the statistics, there may be as many as 12 million cancer diagnoses each year in dogs and cats. Less common, but still significant, are diagnoses in other animals, such as cows, horses, snakes, birds, and fish. Yes, even fish need surgery to remove tumors that can grow from their skin, just like humans.

Cancer types can mimic each other across species. This has allowed veterinary oncology to borrow already-developed human therapies. And it enables cutting-edge research and clinical trials in companion animals to further our understanding of human cancers and provide new therapies to not only benefit those furry family members but also the entire family. An advantage to veterinary clinical trials is the naturally shorter average life spans of companion animals relative to humans. Dr. Wood explains, "Everything is sped up, allowing us to see the accelerated course of the disease and of its treatment to allow us to gain ground faster in the fight against cancer."

Another difference between cancer in humans and companion animals is that pets cannot give voice to when they do not feel well or when something is wrong. Thus the diagnosis of cancer can come at a more advanced stage than in people.

Bottom line—we can learn a lot about human cancers by studying our pets, while also improving the longevity and quality of life for the pets themselves.

Whether it's studying animals, focusing on the disease in laboratories, learning from clinical trials, or evaluating effects on the broad population or its subsets, cancer research has yielded improvement and promises to continue to do so and is, therefore, another reason for hope. But those who actually conduct the research cannot do it alone—they need to be and are supported by a community that enables the progress to be made. We'll look into that community in Chapter 7.

Take a moment to capture your thoughts for this chapter.

1. What are the three key ideas I learned from this chapter?
2. Based on what I learned in this chapter:
   a. What will I want to build into my plans?
   b. Who might help me do this?

Chapter 7

We're Working on It
Research Support

"Someday is Today"
Leukemia & Lymphoma Society

"Get behind a cure"
Fight Colorectal Cancer

Light the Night

In 2015, as part of my consulting work to help the Leukemia & Lymphoma Society develop their strategic plan, I had the opportunity to interview Franklin Smith, MD, who was on the LLS Board of Directors.

Smith is a Pediatric Hematologist-Oncologist, the Vice President for Medical Affairs at Medpace, "a global leader in research-based drug and medical device development," and an Adjunct Professor of Medicine and Pediatrics at the University of Cincinnati College of Medicine, and he had been the Clinical Director of the Cincinnati Cancer Institute at the University of Cincinnati and Director of Hematology/Oncology at Cincinnati Children's Hospital Medical Center.

When I reminded him that I had a vested interest in LLS's success because of my CLL diagnosis, he emphasized the value of LLS funding and of the many researchers and medical professionals who are dedicated to understanding cancers and finding cures. To this day, I recall one thing he said word-for-word, "You know, had you been diagnosed a decade earlier, there was not a good response to CLL."

From September 2014 through January 2015, I had received six rounds of therapy that involved infusions of a combination of Bendamustine and Rituximab (referred to as BR). By all measures, the infusions have been successful. To Dr. Smith's point, Bendamustine had been approved by the FDA as an initial treatment for CLL in 2008, and Rituximab had been approved in 2011.

As I noted earlier, I had agreed to be on a clinical trial, and my arm of the experiment was to receive BR, the currently approved standard of care. Another arm of the trial assessed the performance of an oral drug, Ibrutinib, which had been previously proven effective when used by CLL survivors for whom BR infusions had been unsuccessful. The Ibrutinib arm of the clinical trial I was participating in was testing it as a first-use drug.

The trial was successful. Ibrutinib has been approved by the FDA for first-line use against CLL, making it available for those who will need it in the future.

The reality—I have CLL, as do many others. In 2016, there were about 19,000 new cases diagnosed in the U.S. and about 4,700 died from the disease.

The hope—the mortality rate has significantly improved and continues to do so. And new therapies are being investigated, proven, and deployed as enhanced standards of care.

My hope—continued remission and watchful waiting, every three month visits to Dr. Bartlett for bloodwork and examination.

My pledge—continue to financially support the Leukemia & Lymphoma Society by participating in their annual Light the Night event.

Follow the Money

What does it take to ensure that cancer research continues to improve prevention, detection, diagnosis, and therapy? What does it take to ensure that survivors, regardless of geography or socioeconomic status, have access to the best knowledge and care?

In order to make progress, there must be capable researchers partnering with survivors who are willing to participate in clinical trials. There must be public policy that removes barriers to access. And there must be funds that are raised and allocated to pay for it all.

Let's first follow the money to see where it comes from and where it goes. There are many sources of research funding in the U.S., the four most prominent being the federal government, research fundraising organizations, direct private donations, and the pharmaceutical industry. Importantly, these entities frequently work together to move new therapy discovery and development through the process to bring improved treatments to patients.

1. In 2017, nearly $5.4 billion was budgeted for the National Cancer Institute (NCI), "the federal government's principal agency for cancer research and training." The NCI deploys these funds around the country among the 69 NCI-Designated Cancer Centers at which research is done, and the NCI conducts research itself.

    NCI-funded research is allocated to understand the mechanisms of what causes various types of cancers and what makes them spread, such that therapies can be targeted to specific causes; to learn how to better prevent cancer; to study how to improve detection and diagnosis; to discover and develop new treatment therapies; and to advance general public health as it relates to cancer.

    Among the NCI cancer centers are 49 referred to as Comprehensive Cancer Centers that conduct research, provide services directly to cancer patients, conduct clinical trials (sometimes coordinated across a number of the centers), provide cancer information to health care professionals and the public, and through education, ensure the nation maintains a sufficient cadre of qualified cancer researchers and medical professionals. The vision is that there is an NCI-designated cancer center is within the reasonable proximity of every person living in the country.

    Included in NCI funding is an additional $1.8 billion, to be applied over seven years for the purpose of implementing what is called the "Beau Biden Cancer Moonshot," named for former Vice President Joe Biden's son, who died of brain cancer in 2015. The added spending was authorized in 2016 by the "21st Century Cures Act," with the express objective of making ten years of progress in five years.

2. There are numerous organizations that raise money for research and survivor services. Among them are the American Cancer Society and the Prevent Cancer Foundation that address a range of cancer types.

And there are cancer-specific organizations, like Breast Cancer Foundation, American Childhood Cancer Organization, Fight Colorectal Cancer, and American Lung Association.

These organizations rely on donors either to contribute directly or to participate in fundraising events. For example, when I referred to Light the Night earlier in the chapter, I was speaking of an annual event coordinated to be held around the country. Individuals and teams raise money for LLS, which allocates about $50 million each year to fund nearly 300 blood cancer research projects. You can refer back to the Beat AML Master Trial in Chapter 6 as but one example.

3. Cancer research institutions also receive contributions directly from donors. Frequently, these donors are "grateful patients" in recognition of the therapy they received that had been developed by the research community. The benefactors may also be families of patients who have died, but who still want to acknowledge the care their loved one received and to help ensure that no other family goes through the same ordeal in the future.

In 2004, Otto Ruesch, a prominent businessman and philanthropist, died of pancreatic cancer at the age of 64. He had been treated at the Lombardi Comprehensive Cancer Center on the campus of Georgetown University in Washington D. C. Through a generous gift from Ruesch's wife, Jeanne, Lombardi was able to create the Otto J. Ruesch Center for the Cure of Gastrointestinal Cancers. She says, "Through the course of Otto's illness, we saw so many families whose suffering touched our hearts and made us feel that we had to take some responsibility for trying to make a difference in treating this terrible disease."

Certainly not every donation is as substantial as the Ruesch gift, but each one is as heartfelt and generous and can be applied to support needed research.

4. The only one of these four prominent cancer research funders that is for-profit is the pharmaceutical industry. There are many who critique the industry for being more profit-driven than patient-

centered and for designing and conducting studies that are influenced by conflicts of interest. That being said, the industry does provide support for investigator-initiated clinical trials at academic medical centers, where the specific study is designed, conducted, and controlled by the respective principal investigator. Despite which side of the controversy you are on, it is a fact that the collective industry is a dominant funder of cancer research.

The trends indicate that the number of clinical trials funded by companies is on the rise, while the number funded by government sources is declining.

Revisiting Robbie

Lou DeGennaro, PhD, is President and Chief Executive Officer of the Leukemia & Lymphoma Society and is proud to declare that LLS remains true to the basis upon which Rudolph and Antoinette de Villers founded the organization in 1944 to honor their son, Robbie, who had died of leukemia. Their original intent, which remains the focus to this day, was to raise funds to support research to find cures and to help needy patients.

On the patient-assistance front, in 2017 alone, about $70 million went directly to support those in need with support services like the ones you learned of in Chapter 5. And when the rash of devastating hurricanes hit Texas, Florida, and the Caribbean, LLS earmarked an additional one million dollars to help blood cancer survivors, whose lives had been so dramatically affected, replenish lost drug supplies and help them get to treatments.

On the research front, over its 70+ year history, LLS has allocated more than one billion dollars of research funding, importantly, with measureable results. In 2017, for example, the FDA approved 18 new blood cancer therapies, 15 of which had been touched by LLS funding.

Among the blood cancer treatment breakthroughs in 2017 was the FDA approval of CAR-T therapy. DeGennaro acknowledges the innovative nature of the therapy by referring to it as "Star Wars Medicine." The work that led to the eventual use of CAR-T began in 1998, when LLS began funding work by Dr. Carl June at the University of Pennsylvania. Over nearly two decades, LLS continued its commitment to the promise of the developing science by providing over $21 million.

The result is that children with ALL (Acute Lymphoblastic Leukemia) and adults with CLL, including yours truly, have access to what is proving to be a successful immunotherapy that can be deployed when attempts to manage the disease with previous standards of care have been exhausted.

CAR-T stands for Chimeric Antigen Receptor-T Cells. Remarkably, the approach grew out of Dr. June's research on HIV, the virus that causes AIDS, ultimately leading to a method of engineering a patient's T-cells to trigger the immune system to target specific cancer cells.

The approach is now being tested across a range of other cancer types. Dr. June, for example, is leading a clinical trial to test CAR-T in pancreatic cancer patients. This is but one example of how LLS blood-cancer-focused funding is also affecting cancer therapies broadly.

One aspect of LLS work that was not initially envisioned by the de Villers is that of advocacy. Relatively recently, LLS concluded that research to find cures is absolutely necessary but not sufficient. If cures are available but survivors do not have access to them for any number of reasons, then the therapies are not fully effective. LLS and other organizations have dedicated funding and staff to work with legislators at the state and national levels to establish public policy to ensure everyone has access to available therapies.

A Perfect Fit

There are many non-profit cancer organizations, large and small, that fund research as part of their mission. They are staffed by professionals who profoundly care about that mission and who focus both on raising funds and doing the work.

And those organizations are governed and supported by Boards of Directors, made up of individuals who also care deeply about the mission and who bring diverse expertise to the enterprise. A great example is Ron Doornink and the Fight Colorectal Cancer (Fight CRC) organization, whose mission it is "to empower and activate a community of patients, fighters, and champions to push for better policies and to support research, education, and awareness for all those touched by this disease."

Doornink lost his sister to colon cancer and then lost his brother-in-law to the same disease. His sister's diagnosis at age 37 was fully unexpected, as there was no family history. Doornink's brother-in-law, however, did have a family history, having lost his father to colon cancer. Yet he still chose not to have a colonoscopy, a procedure that would have likely detected his cancer early enough to have saved him. The brother-in-law's death left two orphaned children.

This series of events inspired Doornink's passion to help others prevent, detect, and fight colon cancer, making Fight CRC a perfect fit. Importantly, Doornink brings extensive business and leadership skills and experience to the organization's board.

In Chapter 9, you'll learn more about a life planning tool I call "Finding the Magic." It prompts you to identify your passions, acknowledge your skills, and learn where you can make a difference. When you align your life pursuits with these three things, you have found the magic. This is what Doornink has done such that both he and Fight CRC benefit.

You met Teri Griege earlier—she is the stage IV colon cancer survivor who finished the Ironman. She is passionate about helping others build hope in the face of cancer. She is a skilled and experienced motivational speaker. And she too has found Fight CRC and the needs the organization serves. Teri has also found the magic—another perfect fit.

Win-Win

Mark Kochevar, now retired, had been on the front lines of bringing improved care to cancer survivors since the 1970s, when he began his administrative career at the National Cancer Institute of the National Institutes of Health. After nearly two decades at NCI, he moved on to be Administrative Director at the University of Maryland's Greenbaum Cancer Center, the Associate Center Director at the Medical College of Georgia Cancer Center, and then Associate Director of Administration and Finance at the University of Colorado Comprehensive Cancer Center.

Having lost his father to cancer, Kochevar dedicated his career to the field, and he was especially passionate about one particular aspect, ensuring that every patient has access to the best of care. In his most recent role, for example, he recognized that not everyone in the Colorado region can readily take advantage of the extensive capabilities of the Colorado Cancer Center in Denver.

Although many of the region's remote hospitals administer the standard of care, patients in those areas may not have access to the right specialist for their particular cancer, and they may not have access to cutting edge clinical trials. Kochevar led work to bring capability to those outside the Denver area as well as making sure those who need it can take advantage of the capabilities associated with the Cancer Center.

Although Kochevar's first priority was helping survivors, providing access also created a win-win for the Cancer Center, increasing the size of the pool from which participants can be recruited for critical clinical trials.

Those individuals and organizations that support cancer research and advocate for access add sturdy building blocks to our foundation of hope.

Take a moment to capture your thoughts for this chapter.

1. What are the three key ideas I learned from this chapter?
2. Based on what I learned in this chapter:
    a. What will I want to build into my plans?
    b. Who might help me do this?

Balance

"Life is like riding a bicycle.
To keep your balance, you must keep moving."
Albert Einstein

"I want balance in my life."
Ron Dellums

Life is a Balancing Act

The importance of bringing balance into our lives is not a new concept derived solely from or for our cancer experience. During our school years, we strive to balance attention to our studies with extracurricular activities to enable us to grow intellectually, socially, and emotionally. In our careers, we struggle to create a work/life balance. As parents, we hope to balance giving our children room to explore with the need to keep them safe.

In his 1990 book, *Oh, the Places You'll Go*, Dr. Seuss leads us into our futures with verse after verse of sage advice, which is why the book is a frequent graduation gift. In one verse, Seuss writes,

So be sure when you step.
Step with care and great tact
and remember that Life's
a Great Balancing Act.

If Dr. Seuss wrote it, it must be true.

Our approach to *Balancing Reality and Hope* is to mindfully create and live our cancer and non-cancer plans. We'll acknowledge and act upon the reality that is our cancer and balance that reality with hope. And we'll balance leaning into our future while also living in the moment.

What Happened to Sheila

Sheila Schwartz was an award-winning writer and collegiate creative writing teacher who was diagnosed with ovarian cancer. When she pressed her oncologist for a prognosis, he told her, "You can continue on for quite a number of years."

"What does that mean?" she asked.

"Two? Five? More, perhaps," he responded.

Eight years, two remissions and a third return later, Sheila was still planning for her future when she died. In his article, "What Happened to Sheila," that he wrote after her death, her husband, Dan Chaon, reflected, "...we continued to make plans. We went stepping gingerly into the future, expectantly. It seems crazy now that I look at the credit card bill, but we made plane reservations for a trip to Europe a year in advance. We worried over the flower garden, getting it ready for the winter so that it would be pretty when the spring came. Sheila spent hours alone in her study, finishing the novel that she wouldn't live to see published, and she began to schedule readings and so forth. On her computer were outlines of two new books of short stories, elaborate notes and drafts and tables of contents."

Sheila Schwartz is a role model for *Balancing Reality and Hope*. Despite having a relatively short hope horizon, she leaned into her future, investing her energy to live in the moment and take action day-to-day. She took treatment action opting for surgery and chemotherapy. She took family action, continuing to care for her three young children. She took passion action, working on her writing and traveling and gardening. And when it was the right time, she took action by opting for hospice care.

What would her post-diagnosis life have been and how long would it have been had she not acknowledged reality but only had hope? What if she merely accepted reality but had no hope? But Schwartz had both and balanced them well—living longer than most with late stage ovarian cancer, and living the best life she could for eight years, day-to-day and year-to-year. It's the balance that made the difference.

"...and remember that Life's a Great Balancing Act."

Planning

"Life is what happens to you while you're busy making other plans."
John Lennon (Allen Saunders)

"May your choices reflect your hopes, not your fears."
Nelson Mandela

Planning is a fundamental element of creating and living a balanced life. Whether you do it formally or not, consciously or not, you've been planning all your life. As you progressed through school, you planned to get assignments done, to study for tests, to go to school sports and social events, and to attend parties with friends.

During your working years, you planned to get tasks completed, to develop business plans, to create lesson plans—virtually every occupation requires some level of planning. During those same years, you may have planned a family, kept a detailed calendar to get the children to their activities and get you to meetings and social engagements, and planned for life cycle events like births, graduations, and weddings.

You may have developed a financial plan, planned home improvement projects, and planned vacations. You may be retired and have a plan for how you want to spend your precious time in this new life chapter—perhaps balancing your own activities with those of your grandchildren and other family members.

You get the point—planning has been a big part of your life, whether you have done it mindfully or ad hoc. Now that you or a loved one is a cancer survivor, you've entered a new life stage.

It's a critical stage in which mindful planning can help ensure you have everything lined up to address reality and build hope. In these final two chapters, you'll have the opportunity to develop both your cancer plan and your non-cancer plan—and to do so with intention.

Before we dive in, let's take a look at planning in general.

Punched in the Mouth

Former undisputed heavyweight boxing champion, Mike Tyson, was once billed as the "Baddest Man on the Planet." Although not thought of as the most insightful, articulate guy around, something Tyson said fits well with where we are in our thinking about *Balancing Reality and Hope*, "Everybody has a plan, until they get punched in the mouth."

We had a plan for our lives before our cancer diagnosis punched us in the mouth. It's time to put our next plan together. Might we get punched in the mouth again? Yes. Is that a reason not to have a plan? No, quite the opposite.

Earlier in the book, we gained insight about hope from Shane Lopez, and we can also learn from him about the value of planning. He wrote, "If we have a vision and plan for the future, we can't help but be pulled forward by life, even when our present betrays us...As we fill in more details and take small steps in our future direction, our energy is freed up. When we're excited about 'what's next,' we invest more in our daily life, and we can see beyond current challenges."

Another perspective comes from Doctors Steven Southwick and Dennis Charney. For their book, *Resilience: The Science of Mastering Life's Greatest Challenges*, they reviewed existing studies and interviewed people who seemed to be most resilient. Among them were former Vietnam War POWs, Special Forces instructors, and others from many walks of life. Their research enabled them to identify what they refer to as "resilience factors."

One of the common themes they discovered among these high-resilience individuals is realistic optimism, a belief in a brighter future. This is not about being optimistic regardless of the circumstances—it is not about blind optimism. Rather it is about acknowledging reality and using the information you have to set a course toward the best possible outcome. Realistic optimism is about deliberately planning for and then believing in that brighter future.

Southwick and Charney also contend that being resilient, bouncing back, is a choice. They acknowledge there are those of us who have sufficiently serious conditions that make it more difficult to bounce back; there are those of us who are more predisposed than others to be capable of doing so; and there are those whose life circumstances (such as financial security, relationships, and education) enable us to be more resilient. But all that being said, each of us can make a choice to be more resilient. And we can make a choice to be mindful about our planning.

With that in mind, let's build our plans to help "see beyond current challenges," to envision and create "our brighter future," and to help us stay the course even if we get "punched in the mouth."

Planning Principles

Having worked for the Procter & Gamble Company for 33 years, I learned a lot about the importance to the success of a business of investing the energy to follow some key tried-and-true planning principles. Fortunately, the value of planning and the key principles extend beyond business into our daily lives. Knowing this, I began developing my retirement life plan several years before I retired and in doing so, was able to transition smoothly and with confidence.

In retirement, I've continued to apply the basic planning principles both for me personally and to help others. As I mentioned in the "Introduction," I've had the opportunity to facilitate strategic planning for large cancer organizations and smaller local nonprofits. And as an author (www.aaspector.com), two of my books have focused on helping others plan for the non-financial aspects of their retirement lives.

The planning principles I learned at P&G and the concepts and tools in my retirement planning books have stood the test of time. Since *Your Retirement Quest* was published in 2010, coauthor and friend, Keith Lawrence, and I have been pleased with the book's ongoing value to readers, and we continue to be asked to conduct workshops around the country. These principles, concepts, and tools are the foundation of how you and I will approach life planning in these next two chapters.

To be clear, it is not my intention to suggest you spend your whole life planning your life. Rather, it is to provide you with some simple, yet useful, concepts and tools that will minimize your investment of time while prompting your thinking and having the greatest positive effect.

We'll start with the principles for you to keep in mind as you develop your plans. They are listed and described in no particular order of importance. They all apply.

Don't Wait

Depending on your diagnosis, you may not have the wherewithal, at least initially, to focus on anything but your cancer plan. That being said, a common mistake people make in planning is to fall into the trap of saying, "I'll figure it out later."

Certainly don't wait to ensure your cancer plan is as thorough as it needs to be. And don't wait any longer than you must to develop your non-cancer life plan. The risk is that you'll get into a narrow comfort zone, or for some of us a discomfort zone, which will make it difficult to pursue what's possible. Get started as soon as you are able to create and live the best life you can.

Be Mindful; Be Intentional

There is value in spontaneity—sometimes it's just plain fun to do something on a whim, and you should take advantage of those times when possible. However, if that's all you do, you may be missing opportunities to mindfully plan to do things that will have a positive impact on your future and have the most meaning to you.

The tools in these two chapters will help you approach your planning with intention. Put those plans in place—then add the spontaneity. Great combination.

Focus on What You Can Control

Recall that one of the components of our model for building hope is, "Control What You Can; Create a Plan." We acknowledged that even before our cancer diagnosis, we could not control everything about our lives, but there were things we could control.

For example, we can't control what the stock market does, but we can control how we invest our assets. We can't control the price of goods and services, but we can develop a budget and control how we spend our money. We can't always control who our work colleagues are, but we can control who our friends are. We can't control the vast majority of issues plaguing our community, but we can control where we spend our time to volunteer on the issues about which we are most passionate.

Going forward, two of your most precious resources are your time and energy. Wouldn't it be best to spend them wisely on things you can control?

Focus on What's Important to You

When the late neurosurgeon, Paul Kalanithi, was diagnosed, he struggled to figure out how to best spend what remained of his life, given what would likely be a severely shortened hope horizon. Should he focus on returning to the medical career he had worked so hard to develop, on spending more time with family, on writing a book, or on something else on his list?

When he was discussing this dilemma with his oncologist, she provided this advice, "You have to figure out what's important to you."

Good advice for her patient and good advice for us. In fact, it's good advice whether you are a survivor, loved one, or even someone who is not touched by cancer. Regardless of our personal hope horizon, our precious time and energy would be best spent on that which is important to us.

Stretching and Realistic

The reality is that your cancer diagnosis may impose restrictions on your ability to do everything in your life you want to do. Depending on the level of those limitations, the non-cancer part of your life may be substantial or less so.

Regardless of the severity of the constraints, the principle of stretching and realistic still applies. As we've said frequently throughout the book, we need to acknowledge the reality of the effects of the disease and its treatment. Yet we can also benefit by stretching ourselves to create our best life.

This is not about creating goals or plans that are overwhelming and unattainable. Rather, it is about getting out of our comfort zone without striving for the impossible. That's why the words "stretching" and "realistic" should be thought about together as we plan.

Planning is a Team Sport

There is a risk that our cancer diagnosis causes us to be, or at least feel, isolated, either as the survivor or caregiver. An additional risk is assuming the attitude, "I'll figure it out myself."

That's why you'll build a support team as part of the planning process. Not only can your teammates support your plans, but they can also help you build those plans.

Write it Down

You are more likely, some say five times more likely, to actually live your plan if you write it down. As you go through these next two planning chapters, you'll find descriptions of simple forms you can use. Whether you use the forms or create your own or whether you actually write or create a computer document, you're ahead of the game.

Review and Renew

Who knows better than cancer survivors and their loved ones that life circumstances change? When those circumstances change, your plan may need to change.

Normally, when we think about changing life circumstances, we tend to think of bad things that can happen. But there are positive changes as well, and they too sometimes require a change in plans. You go into remission. Your oncologist tells you you're "cured." You become a new parent, aunt, grandfather. A promising new clinical trial becomes available.

When meaningful changes occur, whether positive or negative, it's prudent to review your plan and renew it as appropriate.

Skill, Will, and Support

Creating your plan is one thing—actually doing it is another. It's possible that your plan will include things you need to change in your life, and making change can be difficult. For example, do you have any New Year's resolutions you still haven't gotten to? Don't we all?

One approach to more successfully make life changes is to put three things in place: 1) acquire the necessary skill/knowledge to do what you want to do; 2) demonstrate the will to make the change; "and" (not "or") 3) recruit support to help you hold yourself accountable to make the change.

Skill—part of the model to build hope urges you to "build your knowledge" about your cancer and its treatment options. Doing so makes you more capable of actively participating in making decisions and taking action with regards to your cancer plan. The same holds true for your non-cancer life plan.

As an example, perhaps before you were diagnosed, you were a recreational jogger. You aspire to return to running the roads, but you may not be able to do so for a while. One of the reasons you had been running was the enjoyment of the outdoors, and you'd like to replace running with another outdoor activity that is less strenuous. For some time, you've been admiring your neighbor's landscaping and surmise you would enjoy doing some gardening on your property, but you know little about what to do. First step—build some basic knowledge and skill. You can't do it if you don't know how.

Will—making the personal commitment to make the change comes in two parts: 1) taking the first steps as soon as possible, and 2) staying the course for a reasonable period of time. In our gardening example, perhaps the first steps are to select a small area in which to start and to purchase some basic gardening tools. In fact, this pertains to another principle, so let's cover it here.

Be Specific—in your planning, be as specific as you can about what you want to do. If your plan reads, "Be a gardener," that doesn't tell you what to actually do next. But if it says, "Buy garden tools" and "Select a bed to begin," you will know what to do. Once those first steps are complete, you can update your plan to the next specific steps.

Then build gardening time into your calendar (yes, write it down), perhaps two-to-three times per week, working your schedule around doctor appointments, treatments, and other life activities. Once you've done the new thing in your life consistently-some say it takes about three weeks-it will more likely become part of your routine and enjoyment.

If you find, after getting this far along, that you really don't enjoy the activity, there is no reason to feel disappointed. You ran an experiment and learned something. Time to revise your plan with something else that promises to be meaningful for you.

Support—some of us have the self-discipline to decide to do something and just do it. But I suspect you know more people who do not have that discipline than those who do. Back to gardening—perhaps you could recruit your neighbor to come over each week, so you can show her your progress. You'll feel more accountable to following your plan—just knowing she's coming will help keep you on track. And, by the way, when she's there, she'll likely have some tips (further building your knowledge) and provide encouragement.

Voila—you're a gardener!

Keep Skill/Will/Support in mind as you proceed, regardless of what your plans turn out to be. It's applicable whether it pertains to your cancer or non-cancer plans.

OK—are you ready to apply these principles and develop your plans?

Chapter 8

Your Cancer Plan

"She stood in the storm and when the wind did not blow her way,
she adjusted her sails."
Elizabeth Edwards

"Today you are you, that is truer than true.
There's no one alive who is youer than you."
Dr. Seuss

Priority One

Priority One: address your cancer with a plan that will achieve the best possible outcomes.

Your plan will include what you decide to do and who will support you along the way. This chapter's intent is to provide you with planning tools to make best use of what you've learned from your medical team, from your own research, and from what you've gleaned from the book thus far.

Planning applies both to you as a survivor and to you as a loved one. You may want to develop a single plan for everyone to follow, or you may find it helpful for each to have his or her own plan. How you approach it may depend on who the survivor is. If the survivor is a child or an aging senior, for example, loved ones may play a more involved planning role.

Crucial Conversation Alert

The opportunity is for survivor and loved ones to collaborate to make sure the plans are all they can be and to make sure that everyone is aligned with each other's plans.

Here's a non-cancer-related example that emphasizes the need to have the crucial conversations. I was conducting a workshop helping people think about planning for the non-financial aspects of retirement. To get the session started, I asked each person to tell the group who they were and why they were there. A gentleman stood and said, "My name is Charles Smith. I'm planning on retiring in three months and want to learn what I need to be thinking about."

The good news was that he was engaging in the planning process for retirement. The bad news was that the woman next to him shouted, "You're what?"

Yes, it was his wife, and it was the first time he had mentioned to her that he was planning on retiring. Do you think they had had the crucial conversations? The other good news is that by the time the workshop had ended, they were on the same page and had begun the discussions.

Examples of crucial conversations relevant to the cancer plan might be discussions with your oncologist and with the practitioner of a complementary health approach about treatment options, discussions with loved ones and your doctors about criteria for when resuscitation is appropriate and when not, or a discussion with your family about the advisability of traveling to another location to access a clinical trial.

Have the crucial conversations. Align the plans.

Phases

As you transition through survivorship, you may find it helpful to think about recognizing which of these three phases you are in for the purpose of developing your cancer plan.

1. Diagnosis to Treatment—during this phase, you are coming to grips with the reality of the diagnosis, both physically and emotionally. You are focusing on learning as much as you can and working with your doctor to decide on the treatment plan that is best for you. You may be dedicated to getting ready for your conventional medicine standard-of-care but may also be learning and deciding about supportive care and complementary health approaches. You are

deciding who to tell and how to tell them, and you are amassing your support team.

2. Treatment—during this phase, you are adhering to your treatment regimen and adjusting your plan to account for side effects, whether anticipated or not. You may be expanding your support team.

3. Post-Treatment—during this phase, you are assessing the success of the treatment and settling in to what may be a new normal for you. Depending on your prognosis, you may be beginning a short or long-term period of remission or cure, or you may be addressing the reality of a shorter hope horizon. And still you may be expanding your support team.

It is possible that you will cycle through phases 2 and 3 if, for example, you are in remission after treatment but the cancer returns. You may even experience phase 1 again if you are diagnosed with what is referred to as a "secondary cancer." Breast cancer survivors, for example, have a slightly higher risk for certain other types of cancers, like salivary gland, colon, or ovarian cancer.

Recall that I learned that my CLL makes me more prone to skin cancer, and on one of my more frequent visits to my dermatologist, he diagnosed a spot on my neck as a basal cell carcinoma—phase 1.

Some of the things in your cancer plan may be constant across all three phases. You may, for example, retain the same oncologist throughout your survivorship. You may change your diet in response to your diagnosis, then continue that nutritional plan throughout.

Other plan elements may change. The most obvious is that your conventional medicine treatment may begin and end, whether it be a surgical procedure, chemotherapy, radiation, or a bone marrow transplant. You may choose a supportive care approach to address pain but find over time that you no longer need it.

Responding to changing circumstances both between and within the phases will enable you to continue to have the right cancer plan in place.

A Planning Tool

Consider the simple, yet effective, planning tool on page 127. I know from my experience working with pre-retirees to develop their retirement life plans that not everyone reading this book will actually create and write down their plan. Certainly, the choice is yours, but I also know that writing your plan will make it more likely you'll think through it more thoroughly and be more likely to follow it. This tool gives you the opportunity to do both.

Modify the chart to suit your needs. If you want to think about your plan in phases, fill in your current phase in the first row. I've filled in a number of cells in the "Plan Category" column, but certainly add other categories to make sure you fully capture all of the elements of your plan and break down the categories into whatever details make sense for you.

These are some additional categories that might be pertinent to you:

➢ Clinical Trial—this segment of your plan would not only capture the medical aspects of the trial but may also entail some practical considerations. For example, the trial that you decide upon may be at a facility to which you need to travel.

➢ Adherence—recall that some people have difficulty adhering to their treatment plan. What plans might you need to ensure you follow yours?

➢ Psychosocial—might you need professional help addressing issues you are having coping with the emotions of your diagnosis, prognosis, and treatment?

➢ Logistics—depending on your personal situation, you may need to work out transportation and other practical matters, such as grocery shopping, preparing meals, picking up prescriptions, and doing basic housework.

In the chart's medical categories, you may choose to include treatments and their schedules, medications including dosages, and perhaps questions you want to investigate further. For other categories, determine what is most helpful for you. The key is to write the plan details with enough specificity to ensure that when you look at your plan, it will clearly remind you of the things you need to attend to and when. Having it written down also enables your loved ones to see the plan and help you follow it as needed.

Also note that your plan will likely change over time. Revisit it periodically to make sure you've kept it up to date. Perhaps you've moved to a different phase. Perhaps your cancer has changed in either the right or wrong direction. Perhaps you've determined that a complementary or conventional health approach is no longer working and you want to investigate others. Medication dosages may change. When you modify your plan, change the date in the upper right-hand corner to help you know that the plan is current.

As you formulate this plan, you may also want to review the notes you've been taking in the previous chapters to help make sure you've thought of everything.

Note that I've also included a place to keep a diary. I've intended it to be a medical diary, but many people benefit from frequent journaling, and you can use this format to do that as well. I have a medical diary that I started when I was first diagnosed, but it now includes every doctor's visit, for example, those associated with my hip replacements, annual physicals, ophthalmology and dermatology appointments, and changes in medication. Every time I update the medical diary, I make sure my wife has a copy so that she has the record if needed.

I then review my diary before each doctor's visit to make sure I have the right questions ready for him or her and that I can share what else may have happened since seeing them last, including interactions with other doctors. In this way, the diary enables me to coordinate my care across physicians.

In the "Notes" column of the diary, you may want to consider including who the physician or other professional was that you saw, where the appointment was, what tests were run, what the results were, who was with you, what you heard, how you felt, whether and for when you scheduled the next appointment, and anything else you think will be useful for future reference. This is for your use, so include what you believe is going to be most helpful.

Phase: Date:	
Plan Category	**Plan Details**
Conventional Medicine	
Supportive Care	
Complementary Approaches	
Financial Planning	
Diary	
Date	**Notes**

As your cancer plan is unfolding, it will begin to inform you who you will want on your support team. We'll spend some time later in the chapter on building that team.

Care and Follow-Up

In 2006, the Institute of Medicine, the National Research Council, the National Academy of Sciences, and the National Academy of Engineering collaborated to form the Committee on Cancer Survivorship: Improving Care and Quality of Life. They focused the study on those who had completed their primary treatment regimen and were transitioning to the post-treatment phase.

The resulting 534-page report (you're right, I didn't read the whole thing), entitled "From Cancer Patient to Cancer Survivor; Lost in Transition," included a number of recommendations, the second of which read, in part, "Patients completing primary treatment should be provided with a comprehensive care summary and follow-up plan that is clearly and effectively explained. This 'Survivorship Care Plan' should be written by the principal provider(s) who coordinated oncology treatment."

There are three phrases in this recommendation that can inform your cancer plan:

- ➢ "a comprehensive care summary and follow-up plan" –emphasizes the value of documenting both what has transpired and the plan going forward
- ➢ "should be written" –is consistent with our principle that you are more likely to actually do your plan if it is written down

  > Note: There are other advantages of writing your plan versus just hoping to keep it straight in your head. One advantage is that it gives you something you can easily share with loved ones to keep them informed, get them on board, and get their thoughts on ways to make your plan even better. Another advantage is that you'll find a written plan to be useful as a way to document your medical history, including diagnosis, treatments, medications, and side effects. As you progress through survivorship, there may be times when having a recorded history will be important, whether it relates to changes in the status of your cancer or perhaps, the advent of other medical issues.

- ➢ "written by the principal provider(s) who coordinated oncology treatment" –having the oncologist write the summary of the care/treatment provided is of great value

Cathy Bradley, PhD, who you met in Chapter 6, was one of a number of reviewers of the 2006 report. She indicates that the documentation of the comprehensive care summary and follow-up plan by oncologists has been spotty, because writing a comprehensive care summary takes a significant amount of extra time, something they don't typically have.

Her observation is supported by data. A study presented at the 2017 Cancer Survivorship Symposium found that nearly 90% of those who had completed treatment did not receive a Survivor Care Plan, and 65% of those felt one would have been helpful. Not surprisingly, another study surveyed hospital cancer programs and found that only just over one-third felt confident the requirement could be met.

If you feel a care summary and follow-up plan would be helpful, here's an approach that may work for you to ensure you have the information you need:

1. Ask your oncologist to write the comprehensive care summary and follow-up plan.
2. If he or she does so, make sure you understand it.
3. If he or she does not, one approach is to ask for a printout of your treatment history from your electronic medical records. If you've had multiple providers, such as surgery, chemotherapy, and radiation, and their reports reside separately, ask for printouts from each physician.
4. Write your own summary to suit your needs and include your understanding of your follow-up care plan. Ask your oncologist to review it.

Prevention and Early Detection

It is not unusual to think about cancer prevention and early detection only as what we can do to keep from getting the disease in the first place or to detect it early enough to decrease its severity. Prevention steps include things like not using tobacco products in any form, maintaining a healthy weight, exercising regularly, using sunscreen, and paying attention to whether there are potentially harmful ingredients in the food we eat. Early detection examples include mammograms, colonoscopies, and prostate exams at recommended frequencies.

Jan Bresch is the Executive Director of Special Love, a children's cancer charity. She is the former Executive Vice President and Chief Operating Officer of the Prevent Cancer Foundation, whose objective is to "Stop Cancer Before It Starts!—saving lives across all populations through cancer prevention and early detection."

Bresch says that prevention and early detection are right for survivors as well, but, she points out, some survivors are put off by this suggestion of prevention, because they react to it as an accusation that they could have prevented their cancer, and not doing so is their fault.

Consistent with our ongoing theme of *Balancing Reality and Hope...*

Reality—regardless of whether we did everything possible to prevent our cancer or detect it early, the cancer is our reality, as is the risk of recurrence and of secondary cancers.

Hope—following our model of building hope, we can learn from our medical team more about how we can take a survivorship prevention and early detection approach.

Balance—with regard to the recurrence risk, we can build an ongoing surveillance regimen into our post-treatment cancer plan; and with regard to the risk of secondary cancers, we can make lifestyle changes to minimize risky behaviors for prevention and include screening for early detection.

As you include surveillance and screening in your cancer plan, work with both your oncologist and your personal care physician to determine who should be doing what and when—and confirm how they will share findings with each other.

All that being said, just a gentle reminder that prevention and early detection fully applies to caregiving loved ones as well. Would it not behoove each of us to understand the steps we can personally take to prevent cancer, or at the very least, make sure we detect it as early as possible, when it is most treatable?

Genetic Testing

One question you may choose to ask your doctor is whether conducting a genetic test of your cancer cells would help determine your best treatment plan. Another is whether it would be helpful to see a genetic counselor to help you understand the implications of the results. Only lately has this become an available topic of conversation. But recent and ever-increasing advances in what some refer to as personalized, precision, or targeted medicine have made it pertinent.

The general concept is that many of today's therapies attack both cancer and non-cancer cells, causing problems with side effects. But what if your doctor and you knew the specific genetic mutation that caused your cancer, and what if there were a specific treatment that uniquely targeted that mutation? Genetic testing is becoming faster and more affordable, is enabling research advances, is leading to the discovery of targeted therapies, and is enhancing both prevention and diagnostic capabilities.

Targeted medicine has the promise of breakthroughs in the future, but we can already see the value of genetic testing in certain circumstances. Dr. Allison Kurian, Director of the Stanford Women's Clinical Cancer Genetics Program, says, "Why should they (female breast cancer survivors) be getting it (genetic testing)? There are many reasons, but maybe the most important is that for a breast cancer patient, if she has a genetic mutation in BRCA1 or 2, she has a high risk of ovarian cancer that could kill her. When we don't test these patients and we don't find those mutations, we basically miss a chance to save lives."

Another reason for genetic testing for breast cancer survivors is to guide treatment. If positive for BRCA1 or 2, there is an increased risk of cancer recurrence after preliminary treatment, thereby perhaps indicating a choice of mastectomy versus lumpectomy or a choice to have a prophylactic oophorectomy, the surgical removal of one or both ovaries.

Even with these known benefits of genetic testing, it is not as widely used as you might expect. In a study reported in February 2017 in the *Journal of the American Medical Association*, Dr. Kurian and others assessed over 2,500 women who had been diagnosed with stages 0 to II breast cancer. About 30% of the study participants had a higher than average risk of a genetic mutation. Risk was assessed based on family history factors associated with an increased likelihood: if a family member had been diagnosed with breast cancer before age 50, if there have been multiple breast cancers in the family, if there have been both breast and ovarian cancers in the family, and if the family has Ashkenazi Jewish heritage.

The women were surveyed two months after surgery. Of those study participants with high risk, about 80% wanted genetic testing and about 70% talked to a doctor about testing. Yet fewer than 55% received genetic testing. "My doctor didn't recommend it" was the primary reason for those wanting testing not being tested.

One other statistic from the study—of those high-risk women who were tested, just over 60% also met with a genetic counselor. The guidelines of the National Comprehensive Cancer Network (NCCN) indicate that each woman genetically tested should have the benefit of such a session to best understand the test and its results. One issue is that the number of genetic counselors is not keeping up with those guidelines.

As you develop your cancer plan, ask, "Would seeing a genetic counselor and being tested help determine the best treatment plan for my particular cancer?" Then, "Why or why not?"

Beginner's Nerves

In her book, *Dying: A Memoir*, Cory Taylor, the award-winning Australian author, answered questions she has been asked since being diagnosed with stage IV melanoma-related brain cancer in 2005 and learned that her cancer was incurable. Among those questions, "Are you scared?" Taylor wrote,

> *"Yes, I'm scared, but not all the time. When I was first diagnosed, I was terrified. I had no idea that the body could turn against itself and incubate its own enemy. I had never been seriously ill in my life before; now, suddenly, I was face to face with my own mortality. There was a moment when I saw my body in the mirror as if for the first time. Overnight my own flesh had become alien to me, the saboteur of all my hopes and dreams. It was incomprehensible, and so frightening I cried.*
>
> *"'I can't die,' I sobbed. 'Not me. Not now.'*
>
> *"But I'm used to dying now. It has become ordinary and unremarkable, something everybody, without exception, does at one time or another. If I'm afraid of anything, it's of dying badly, of getting caught up in some process that prolongs my life unnecessarily. I've put all the safeguards in place. I've completed an advance health directive and given a copy to my palliative-care specialist. I've made it clear in my conversations, both with him and with my family, that I want no life-saving interventions at the end, nothing designed to delay the inevitable. My doctor has promised to honor my wishes, but I can't help worrying. I haven't died before, so I sometimes get a bad case of beginner's nerves, but they soon pass."*

Cory Taylor died on July 5, 2016, at the age of 61.

If you were diagnosed at age 85, you may have already been thinking deeply about your mortality. If you were diagnosed in your 30s, death may have been the farthest thing from your mind. If your child has been diagnosed, the thoughts may be unfathomable.

If you have a choice, you will not likely build death into your cancer plan. Many will die "with" the disease, not "of" it. Others will be "cured." For others, the prognosis may not be good.

Your diagnosis/prognosis could also be thought about as a wakeup call to do some things that are a good idea anyway. Taylor referred to a "health directive." Do you have one in place and does your family know where to find your will, health and other powers of attorney, bank accounts, trusts, investment and tax documentation, insurance policies, and any other estate interests?

Have you made all of your relevant wishes clear? Doing so will help make sure everyone who needs to has heard them from you and will reduce the risk that there will be decision-making conflicts within the family.

Have you made arrangements for your funeral? It may sound depressing, but making these plans has two benefits. You will know that your preferences will be honored, for example, where you want to be buried. And you will know that at a time that will be heavy with emotion, your loved ones will not need to worry about attending to those details.

Have you accomplished any unfinished goals you find meaningful? Have you made peace in any relationships you'd like to tend to? Have you made arrangements for palliative or hospice care for when you need it? Have you thought about saying your last loving good-byes when that time comes? Have you arranged for pastoral counseling?

Have you gotten answers to your satisfaction to the question, "What will happen when I'm actually dying?"

Have you, to your satisfaction, answered the question, "How do I want to die?"

Attending to these aspects of dying can certainly be an integral part of your cancer plan.

Helpful Services

"Because hospice deals with death, people tend not to talk about it."

So wrote American humorist and prolific Pulitzer Prize-winning author Art Buchwald in his 2006 autobiography *Too Soon to Say Goodbye*.

But let's talk about it, which, by the way, has become more acceptable since Buchwald's book was published a few months before he died at age 81. And talking about it is enormously more acceptable since Dame Cicely Saunders created the first modern hospice in a London suburb in 1967 and since the first U.S. hospice was founded in Branford, Connecticut in 1974.

Given the choice, most of us would opt not to get to the point where we would need hospice care, but the reality is that at some point, we may need the services, either as a result of our cancer or some other reason. As with other aspects of developing our cancer plan, we should ask ourselves and then talk to our loved ones about taking such a step if it seems that it may become necessary.

We can begin to understand hospice care from a single statement made by the National Hospice and Palliative Care Organization, "At the center of hospice...is the belief that each of us has the right to die pain-free and with dignity, and that our families will receive the necessary support to allow us to do so."

More than half of hospice service days are provided at home, just over 40% in nursing homes, and the remaining at hospice centers and hospitals. Supported by nurses, social workers, home health aides, and others, the services can include managing the survivor's symptoms, including pain, providing drugs, supplies, and equipment, helping the family know how to care for the patient, making periodic visits and always being on call, and providing grief counseling to family and friends.

About 1.5 million patients enroll in hospice care each year as measured by Medicare. Of those, more than 25% are cancer patients, and the average length of service is 70 days.

If you or a loved one has likely six months or less to live, you are qualified for hospice care. When you're ready, you can contact a hospice care provider, who will contact your doctor to confirm it's appropriate and then begin to coordinate care. Or you can work directly with your doctor or supportive oncology resources to help you enter the process.

Some people for whom hospice care is part of their cancer plan choose to wait until death is imminent or perhaps days or weeks away. That is certainly a choice you can make, but consider that doing so may not be taking full advantage of the helpful services available for both survivor or loved one.

Lift You Higher

You've likely been part of many teams over the years, whether they were sports teams, work groups, military units, organization committees, or others. In doing so, you have learned the value of a team. Helen Keller said, "Alone we can do so little; together we can do so much." Oprah Winfrey opined, "Surround yourself with only people who are going to lift you higher."

There is no better way to get things done than to create a team of individuals who have a common objective. As a cancer survivor or a loved one, your team's objective should be clear—address the cancer in a way that enables you to live your best life.

You've begun to think about the wide range of things to consider for your cancer plan. It would be additionally helpful to identify and recruit a team to support you—a team that shares your objective.

As your cancer plan changes over time, so might your support team, but build your initial team nevertheless—people who will "lift you higher."

Necessary and Sufficient

Consider this two-word concept—"necessary" and "sufficient." You want your support team to be both. You only want those on your team who are necessary and you want your team to be sufficient to meet your needs. This might sound a bit selfish—that's because it is. It is your cancer, so it will be your plan and your team.

Why should your team be comprised of only those who are necessary? Even though you will benefit from support team members, they will also take your time and energy, whether you are the survivor or the caregiving loved one. You don't want to totally shut out family and friends who mean well and want to be involved, but you do want to focus on those who are adding the most value to your cancer plan.

I had each of my hips replaced in 2013, about four months apart. Doing so relieved arthritis symptoms that not only precluded me from continuing to play baseball, one of my passions, but was also seriously affecting my day-to-day life. My wife and I knew that our full focus needed to be on recovery and rehab. She played the role of gatekeeper to minimize visitors, who, with good heart, wanted to come wish me well. For the first four to five weeks following each surgery, Ann made sure only the visitors necessary to my recovery would be allowed, like my home-health nurse and home-visiting physical therapist. When the time was right, she eased the restrictions.

And why should your team roster be sufficient? It might sound trivial, but you wouldn't play a baseball game without a shortstop or appoint an organization committee without a chairperson. In the same regard, if you have an important need to make your cancer plan, or your non-cancer life plan for that matter, be the best it can be, why would you live with a hole in your lineup such that a need remains unmet?

Necessary and sufficient—a winning team.

You are Your Head Coach

The head coach or manager of a sports team needs to make decisions about who to have on his or her team and who should play each position.

You are your head coach. You are developing your cancer game plan, and you're building your team. You must decide which positions to have and who will fill them. Do you need, for example, a nutritionist, financial advisor, cancer coach, driver, massage therapist, clergy member, home health representative, second-opinion oncologist, chemo buddy, and on and on?

When filling your team positions, you may want to think about two overarching criteria. One is their level of competency and experience. The other is their attitude.

Teammates don't necessarily need to be the best at their position, but you want to have confidence they can get the job done and be there for you. Some of your choices may be easy to make based on your past experience. For example, you may want to avail yourself of pastoral counseling, and you have a previous relationship with the clergy at your congregation.

Other positions on your team may be those with which you have less familiarity. For example, you may want to explore complementary healthy approaches to deal with pain or with side effects of treatment, but you have no experience with acupuncture or nutritional supplements or other offerings. Evaluating these practitioners will require research and following up on references—some of which you may do and some you'll need help doing. In any case, you'll want to learn about their skill and experience level before putting them on your team.

Why might the attitude of your teammates be important, even if they can expertly fulfill their roles? There is a long-held belief, supported by recent studies, and I think most of us would agree intuitively, that attitude is contagious, whether that attitude is positive or negative.

Like most great children's book authors, A. A. Milne created stories for children but with adult sensibilities. Winnie the Pooh's friends have distinctive personalities with which we can relate. How would you describe Tigger? Bouncy, happy, positive. How would you describe Eeyore? Down, negative...depressed.

Do you have Eeyores in your life? You might say that having them is fine—sure they drain energy versus create it, and you may have been willing to tolerate that. But now you have cancer, and it's taking your full reserve of energy to face it head on. Can you afford Eeyores on your team?

I'm not suggesting you blatantly cut every Eeyore from your life, but when you mindfully build your support team, each of them is worth considering. And you certainly don't want to add others. Your attitude is critical. Your energy is critical. Attitude is contagious. Hope is contagious.

Thank you, Ms. Winfrey, "Surround yourself with only people who are going to lift you higher."

Team Roster

In the spirit of continuing to write things down, consider creating a simple team roster chart. Doing so will help ensure that you think about all of the team positions, and it will be something you can share with others for their use.

Try a chart that has three columns—label them "Position," "Name," and "Contact Information." If you find there is other information you'd like to include, add columns.

As a way to get organized, think about the team roster by categories. For example, consider your Medical Team, Family/Friends Team, Personal Care Team, Complementary Health Approach Team, Financial/Legal Team, and others as you see fit. Here are some lists of examples to get you started. Select the ones that make sense for your situation, and add to the lists to make them work best for you.

> ➢ Medical Team: you may want to consider the positions of medical oncologist, surgical oncologist, radiation oncologist, palliative care doctor, family doctor, physical therapist, occupational therapist, nurse practitioner, nurse coordinator, psychologist, pharmacist, and genetic counselor.
> ➢ Family/Friends Team: spouse/partner, other close relatives, close friends, a chemo buddy (someone who accompanies you to treatments). You may think that it's not necessary to include these "obvious" people on your team roster, but consider that this list also serves as a contact sheet. A friend who is driving you to an appointment, for example, may need to contact a doctor or your spouse.
> ➢ Personal Care Team: pastoral counselor, social worker, cancer coach (this is a person you can engage to help you navigate through each aspect of dealing with your cancer), transportation support, hospice care representative, and cancer support group leader.
> ➢ Complementary Health Approach Team: there may be any number of practices and practitioners you consider—nutritionist, personal trainer, tai chi instructor, massage therapist, and yoga instructor.
> ➢ Financial/Legal Team—financial advisor, estate planner, accountant, and insurance agent.

There will be people on your team that don't need to appear on your roster. For example, if your treatment includes chemotherapy infusions, those nurse(s) will be on your team, but when you show up, they'll be there, and they may change for each session. Another example is the phlebotomist who draws your blood for testing—he or she is on your team but will be there when you need them. That being said, if you feel the need to be thorough, fill in these positions and add the contact information of that unit at the cancer center.

CareMap

Perhaps you'd prefer to draw a picture of your support team rather than or in concert with filling in a table.

Rajiv Mehta is the Founder and Chief Executive Officer of Atlas of Caregiving, an organization committed to transforming caregiving "through innovative research, practical solutions, and rich collaboration."

One of their practical solutions is called the Atlas CareMap. The idea is to create a drawing (don't worry—you can use stick figures) of who is in your caregiving support network and how they relate to you and to each other. The process maps around the survivor and the primary caregiver to include who cares for each. It also helps analyze relationships among caregivers and includes consideration of the physical distance each support resource is from the survivor.

Using the tool, you can more readily visualize what is likely a complex network of people to help you ensure your caregiving system will meet your needs. Mehta also helps by prompting some questions you might want to ask that would be appropriate whether you actually use the CareMap drawing approach or not:

> ➤ Who are the most important people on your support team? What would happen if one of them became unavailable? Who would step in? Would they be prepared to do so?
>
> ➤ Are various people in your network aware of others they need to know about?
>
> ➤ Are there other family members, friends, or neighbors who can help? What would it take to get them involved?
>
> ➤ Are there important services or professionals currently missing? How could such help be obtained?
>
> ➤ How has the situation changed over time in a way that would change the CareMap? (And I would add, how might the situation change in the future such that we could anticipate support we may need? For

example, how might the support team change as the survivor transitions through the three phases, diagnosis to treatment, treatment, and post-treatment?)

One of the values of the drawing, Mehta has learned from his research and anecdotal information, is that, at times, a survivor was in the role of caregiver when diagnosed. The CareMap could help envision how to meet both sets of needs, that of the survivor and that of the person the survivor was previously supporting.

You can find brief videos at atlasofcaregiving.com to learn how to draw your own CareMap and how to use it once it's drawn. You can also download a "Guide and Worksheets" document to help you complete the drawing of your support network.

The CareMap, like the team roster table, serves the purpose of creating something that the survivor and loved ones can work on together and capture any changes you decide upon. And it can prompt the crucial conversations to make sure everyone understands what the expectations of them are.

Crucial Conversation Alert

Expectations Exchange

Many of your support teammates will not require any special conversation to recruit them—your loved ones and close friends, for example. If you already have a relationship with your clergy, you'll likely not need any more conversation than letting them know of your diagnosis.

But there may be others with whom you will need deeper conversations. Perhaps, for example, you want to consider acupuncture as a complementary health approach to help you manage pain. It is likely you'd want to have a thorough discussion with the practitioner.

One way to think about these conversations is that each is an expectations exchange. You will want to make it clear what expectations you have and will want to learn what the support teammate expects of you.

A close friend might say, "Whenever you need me, just call." It might come out in your expectations exchange that what that really means is, "If you have an emergency, don't hesitate to call, but between work, my three kids, and my aging parents, who I'm helping care for, my schedule is pretty hectic already."

These crucial conversations may not happen right up front. There is a lot on both of your minds, but the expectations should get clear to make sure everyone can fulfill commitments.

You have developed and will continue to renew and revise your cancer plan. You have a support team and will continue to modify that roster as circumstances change. Time to move on to develop the plan for the part of your life that is not cancer.

Chapter 9

Your Non-Cancer Plan

"My goal is to build a life I don't need a vacation from."
Rob Hill Sr.

"Yes, I have cancer and it might not go away,
But I can still have a future because life goes on."
Kris Carr

Quail Hunting

Recall our earlier definition, "Hope is taking action to develop the genuine belief that the future will be better than the present and/or better than should be expected."

And recall that one of the foundational elements of building hope is "Control What You Can; Create a Plan." Doing so gives you confidence and urges you to lean into your future to make it the best it can be.

And recall we learned about Tom Brokaw's multiple myeloma diagnosis in Chapter 1. In his book, *A Lucky Life Interrupted*, he shared his experience over the first year-plus of his survivorship. Although his cancer was painful, his treatments had their expected side effects, and his emotions ebbed and flowed, his outlook is inspirational.

Brokaw and his wife Meredith are friends with Susan and Jim Baker, who had been the U.S. Secretary of State, Secretary of the Treasury, and White House Chief of Staff under two presidents. This friendship and others enabled Brokaw to help us understand the value of leaning into the future to create one that "will be better than the present."

He writes, "The Bakers and the Brokaws have an annual quail-hunting outing with our wives and other friends, so I wanted Jim to know the goal was to get the cancer under control before the birds were out of season. Those kinds of plans kept me focused on the future and better times. Multiple myeloma was now as much a part of my consciousness as days of the week and news of the day."

Brokaw acknowledges the reality of his cancer and has a cancer plan, but he also has a non-cancer life plan that is comprised of many activities about which he cares deeply, including quail hunting with friends.

No, most of us will have neither the desire nor means to go quail hunting, but each of us can take full advantage of creating and living a meaningful non-cancer life.

The Opportunity

Perhaps cancer has given us an opportunity. It's really difficult to think about that statement, but hang in there with me a bit. It is possible that before our diagnosis, we were living our lives but without intention. Life just showed up, and we reacted to it the best we could. But what if our cancer diagnosis causes us to think differently about life?

Amanda George is the founder of thinkaboutyourlife.org. In the introduction to her "Think About Your Life" workbook, she writes, "I was 30 years old when I started my journey with breast cancer. I remember hearing the words 'you have cancer' and my life changed – mostly for the better.

"As I was struggling through surgeries, chemotherapy, and radiation treatment...I thought about my life – a lot."

Said another way, George began living her life with intention. That's the opportunity.

In this, the book's final chapter, we'll investigate what might be the key elements of our best non-cancer life. And we'll look at some simple tools to bring those elements to life.

Key Elements

When Keith Lawrence and I did our research to write *Your Retirement Quest*, we interviewed hundreds of retirees, reviewed retirement-relevant research, and read every retirement book we could get our hands on. In doing so, we were able to identify what we call the "10 key elements of a fulfilling retirement."

Guess what. They turned out to be the key elements for life in general. Not only have we conducted workshops around the country for retirees, we've also done so for 40-somethings, we've had 20-year olds in our sessions; and we've even been asked if we would do our workshop for Boy Scouts. The key elements can work for everybody.

As you review the brief summary of the key element, think about where you are for each one in your life today. We'll then use the tools that follow to give you ways to incorporate your personal assessment for each element into your non-cancer life plan.

To reemphasize—these key elements and the development of a non-cancer plan apply to both survivor and loved ones.

Attitude

Studies indicate that among the general population, those with a positive attitude live longer on average and have a better quality of life than those with a negative attitude. As we've discussed, a positive attitude in and of itself cannot cure cancer, but it can make a difference in the effectiveness of a treatment plan and in the quality of life for survivors and their loved ones.

Another piece of good news is that our attitude is not hard-wired. We can positively affect it to enhance both our cancer plan and our non-cancer plan. Here are but a few suggestions:

> Sincerely practice gratitude
> Balance leaning into your future while enjoying living in the moment
> Surround yourself with those who have a positive attitude, minimizing your time with Eeyores

The very fact that you are thinking about enhancing the non-cancer part of your life and mindfully developing a plan to do so are signs of having a positive attitude.

Connectedness

Studies have shown both the positive quality-of-life and longevity effects of deeply connecting with others. You can approach connectedness in two impactful ways: 1) stay or get involved with networks and communities and 2) create and nurture deep personal relationships.

What networks or communities were you connected with prior to your diagnosis? Were you part of a work group, religious congregation, special-interest club, volunteer project team, organization committee, sports team, card-playing group? Have you stayed connected or can you return?

If you were not previously part of such communities, there is value in choosing one or two to get involved in. You may have already joined a support group as part of your cancer plan. Ask your fellow support group members what other communities they are involved in as one way to get some ideas.

And to the extent you can stay connected with or develop new two-o'clock-in-the-morning friends, the better off you'll be. These are friends, including family members, who you can call without qualms in the middle of the night if you need help, and without question they will be on the way to you and vice versa. Identify your 2:00am friends/family and nurture them.

A corollary to thinking about connectedness is to guard against the risk of isolation. Being fully focused on cancer and its treatment may make it difficult to stay connected. And friends and family, despite their best intentions, may be finding it difficult to figure out when and how to interact.

Giving Back

You might think you are in a better position to be the recipient of volunteer efforts than volunteering yourself. And in some ways you are. But your cancer experience may present the opportunity to enhance your life satisfaction by also giving back to others.

My brother-in-law and colorectal cancer survivor, Harvey Ferdman, recognized that he could help others who had been newly diagnosed. He volunteered to participate in support groups and one-on-one to share his knowledge and experience to support others as they coped with their diagnosis. But your opportunities are certainly not limited to cancer-related activities. Any form of giving back can be satisfying. Recall Bob Miller from

Chapter 1, who, as a survivor, continues to work on Habitat for Humanity projects.

Studies have shown that those who give back gain even more from the experience than those receiving the support. The studies also indicate that the more closely you interact with the recipient of your volunteer effort, the more personally satisfying it is for you.

Passions

Recall that when Sheila Schwartz died eight years after her ovarian cancer diagnosis, she had made plane reservations for a trip to Europe a year in advance (passion: travel), worried over her flower garden, getting it ready for the winter so that it would be pretty in the spring (passion: gardening), was finishing a novel and had outlines of two new books of short stories on her computer (passion: writing), and was actively caring for her three children (passion: family).

What do you love to do? What causes you to lose track of time? What do you love to learn about and share with others? These are your passions.

Were you pursuing them before your cancer diagnosis? Are you pursuing them now? Yes, it may be more difficult or perhaps impossible for the time being, but the passions continue. Have you found another way to pursue them? A couple of years after my CLL diagnosis, I chose to get my hips replaced to relieve the constant soreness from arthritis. I was prepared for the likelihood that the combination of CLL and hip replacement would preclude me from continuing to play baseball, but I was still passionate about the game.

I searched for and found alternative ways to pursue my passion. I coached my grandson's team. I led several community baseball discussions. I volunteered to facilitate a baseball discussion program to promote cognitive stimulation among those who have been recently diagnosed with dementia. And I contemplated writing another book about baseball—my first book is entitled *Baseball: Never Too Old to Play the Game*. Fortunately, I was able to return to the playing field while also continuing to pursue these other baseball-related activities. Whether I would still have been able to play or not, I had baseball on my non-cancer life plan (passion: baseball).

By the way, did you notice how several of my baseball passion activities also enabled me to give back and another combined my passion for baseball with my passion for writing? The key elements frequently interact.

Have you identified your passions and are you pursuing them?

Financial Security

You are likely attending to financial security as part of your cancer plan, making sure you are dealing with its many aspects. You're covering medical costs through insurance and from your own funds, and you may be dealing with the possibility that you'll not be able to work, at least for a while. You're tending to getting financial affairs in order by working with your insurance agent and estate planner as needed.

One way to think about financial security is that these are steps you may have already taken care of prior to your diagnosis. If not, and even if you are happy to find yourself cancer free, these matters deserve your attention.

Financial security is not about the size of your nest egg, but rather about three things: 1) matching your lifestyle and budget to your available resources, 2) having your financial and legal paperwork in place, and 3) ensuring your loved ones are aware of your financial plan.

Life Purpose

In my retirement workshops, I ask attendees to ask themselves the question, "What is my life purpose?" Many people answer that question by declaring the role they play. They view their purpose as being a teacher or a mom or a business owner or whatever role they most relate to. From a retirement perspective, that can be an issue. When you retire or when the children move out of the house, the role that you identified as your purpose is over. How do you then redefine yourself?

In your cancer context, you may have a similar dilemma. Before diagnosis, you may have had a role that you felt defined you. After diagnosis, you may be asking and perhaps dreading the answer to the question, "Does my cancer now define me?"

There are two possible paths to take from here regarding life purpose. One path is to spend the introspective time-perhaps you are doing that already-to get clear about life purpose. The other path is to simplify the question a bit by changing it from "What is my life purpose" to "What can I do with my time that is important?"

The answer may derive from the other key elements—you may choose to pursue a passion, spend time giving back, or maximize your connectedness. Either path will help your quality of life; pick one - or both.

Wellbeing

You may argue that understanding this key element is a no-brainer. Of course, wellbeing means being cancer free, or reducing the cancer to a chronic condition, or making the best of a difficult prognosis, or coping with both the physical and emotional aspects of the disease. And I would agree with you. Regardless of the level of progress you are making, part of your wellbeing can be measured by the state of your cancer.

But that's not the only way to assess whether you have the level of wellbeing you would like. Think about it this way. There are things you want to do in your non-cancer life now and into your future. In order to do them, you will need to have the energy to do so.

In order to develop and sustain that energy, consider doing two things— be true to your cancer plan and adopt the daily habits that build versus drain energy.

These habits may be associated with your physical energy, like exercise, sufficient sleep, proper nutrition. The habits may be associated with emotional energy, like taking steps to relieve stress, practicing gratitude, surrounding yourself with Tiggers versus Eeyores. The habits may be associated with mental energy, like focusing on what you can control, stimulating yourself intellectually, stretching yourself out of your comfort zone. The habits may be associated with energy of purpose, which for some is linked to their faith, and for others it has to do with identifying your life purpose and living to that purpose.

Attending to these daily habits will build energy and help ensure you sustain that energy as best you can into your future, regardless of your hope horizon.

Growth

In the retirement arena, the growth key element pertains to making sure that one stays intellectually stimulated after leaving the primary career. In the cancer arena, I'd suggest growth has a different and broader relevance.

One opportunity to enrich our lives in general, is to continue to grow as human beings, intellectually, experientially, spiritually, socially, emotionally, and physically. Perhaps doing so is even more important after the trauma of a cancer diagnosis.

A term that is getting more use is "post-traumatic growth," which indicates that some people see cancer as an opportunity to reassess their lives and to take action to do what moves them. Studies are showing that those who do so tend to experience less anxiety and exhibit fewer symptoms of depression.

We can't control the reality that we have been diagnosed, but we can develop our cancer and non-cancer life plans to control what we can. The result—to continue to grow as human beings.

There are stories of survivors who have founded major cancer fundraising organizations, who have challenged themselves physically by competing in triathlons for the first time after diagnosis, and who have started businesses. But it doesn't have to be the big audacious accomplishments. What moves you? Is it getting back to work? Is it rearing your family? Is it becoming the veteran member of your support group, helping others like others helped you?

Regardless, it is about controlling what you can to ensure post-traumatic growth.

Fun

Although you can enter "having fun with cancer" into your search engine and find a number of stories of people finding ways to have fun while coping with cancer, this key element is not about that.

What this is about, and perhaps the key element that best exhibits the value of having a non-cancer plan, is finding ways in that segment of your life to just plain have fun. And it is the key element that flies in the face of the value of planning. Fun frequently comes from spontaneity—by definition, unplanned.

But you can be mindful about being open to spontaneous moments. Many of us have our good days and our bad days. On the next good day, pick something to do on a whim and go for it.

If you lived within reasonable driving distance of the world's largest catsup bottle, would you go see it? My brother-in-law, a colorectal cancer survivor, and I, a leukemia survivor, did just that. We added lunch at a local diner, and drove a bit further to take a tour of the Cahokia Mounds State Historic Site. Just plain fun!

Planning

This final key element pulls the others together, and it is the one that we're going to spend time on together, keeping all of the key elements in mind, through the remainder of this chapter. Having a written plan will help you set priorities, hold yourself accountable for doing the things you want to do, and give you a vehicle for having crucial conversations with those closest to you.

Importantly, the non-cancer life plan will complement the cancer plan. Together, they will help you acknowledge your current reality, build hope, and balance the two.

Planning Tools

There are a number of planning tools you can use to prompt you to think about, create, and live your non-cancer plan. Pick the one or ones that would work best for you, but I'd suggest that you at least give each one a try. And remember, there is value in writing down your plan instead of just keeping it in your head.

We'll look at four planning tools and one planning concept in enough detail for you to be able to use them. The four tools are "Bucket Jars," "Finding the Magic," "Your Best Day," and "Making Life Changes," and the planning concept is "Renewal."

Bucket Jars

Yes, that's right—it says "Bucket Jars" and not "Bucket List." There's nothing wrong with a bucket list, so let's look at that a bit before coming back to the jars. I prefer to think differently about a bucket list than it was treated in the 2007 movie, *The Bucket List*, with Morgan Freeman and Jack Nicholson.

In the movie, the main characters, hospital roommates, each with a terminal illness, seek to complete a list of things they want to see and do before they die. There's a more uplifting way to think about bucket lists - and jars - regardless of our diagnosis and prognosis.

Consider it a list of things you are excited about looking forward to doing, about planning to do, about actually doing, about the people with whom you'll do them, about relating your experience to others, about reminiscing afterwards, and about deciding if you want to do them again.

The list can be made up of big dreams like a travel destination, writing a novel, or skydiving. And it can include smaller things, like going to that new neighborhood restaurant, seeing a live performance of that band whose music you love, teaching your granddaughter to play a card game your grandmother taught you, or visiting each of the county parks in your area— smaller in scope but not necessarily in enjoyment.

OK, back to bucket jars. I was interviewing a woman for my retirement life planning book and asked her if she had a bucket list. She said, "No. I have bucket jars. One jar is labeled 'Activities and Games.' A second is 'Let's Eat.' And the third is 'Oh, the Places We'll Go.'"

She continued, "Whenever I hear about something that intrigues me, I write it on a small piece of paper and put it in the right jar. Then when I want to plan something to do, I empty a jar and sort through my notes, pick one, and make plans."

Some of us may not have the wherewithal to take full advantage of bucket jars, but perhaps even for those of us who may be having more bad days than good ones, the planning tool can still make sense. What if you labeled your jars or organized your list by "good days" and "bad days?"

"Good Days" might be for items that are out of the house but close to home, like trying that new restaurant, seeing a movie that just came out, or taking a friend to the park. "Bad Days" might be for items inside the house, but ones that still meet the criteria to fit on your bucket list, primarily things you are really looking forward to doing. These might include getting carry-out from that new restaurant, watching the next episode of your favorite binge series, or inviting a friend over who you haven't seen for a while.

Constantly add to your jars/list as you hear about new possibilities. Even if you're having more bad days than good, you'll be getting in the habit of listing and checking off items—then when things get better, you'll be able to expand your horizons.

Finding the Magic

In many ways, these planning tools are helping you answer the question, "What can I do with my time that is important?" There may be no better method of doing this than "Finding the Magic!"

To find the magic, think about three questions. The first is, "What are my passions?" Or "What do I love to do?"

The second is, "What are my strengths?" Or "What am I good at?"

The third is, "What does my community need?" Or "Who needs my help and with what?"

Answer these questions, then figure out how to spend your time doing something that touches all three, something you are passionate about, that plays to your strengths, and for which there is a need. Once you do, you will have found the magic.

My baseball passion I described earlier is one example. I'm passionate about baseball. I have experience leading group discussions. And there is a need to help those recently diagnosed with dementia stimulate their brains. I volunteered to facilitate the program. Magic!

A friend is passionate about his religious congregation, and he is a building contractor. His congregation's facilities were in need of renewal. He led the effort to refurbish both the interior and exterior of the structure. Magic!

Another friend has long been passionate about children's causes, and she is an educator. She learned of the need to accelerate reading proficiency at a local school. She's tutoring fourth graders. Magic!

Once you figure out where your magic is, schedule your time to make it fit with everything else going on in your life, whether those activities are part of your cancer plan or your non-cancer plan. When you fit it in, you'll find you'll derive a great deal of personal fulfillment. Magic!

Your Best Day

What if every day were your best day, every week your best week, every year your best year?

Because you or a loved one has cancer, you know that there are parts of your days that are affected by that reality and by what you need to do to follow your cancer plan. You may need to spend part of the day in an infusion pod. You may find yourself profoundly fatigued in the middle of the afternoon. You may be recovering from surgery. As a loved one, you may be transporting your family member or friend to a doctor's appointment. You may be checking in with the survivor every morning.

There are a lot of things that can get in the way of living an ideal day in your non-cancer plan. But if you acknowledge the realities and build around them, you should be able to envision your best day.

Again, let's write it down. Create a table with two columns on paper or electronically. In the first column, list times in half-hour increments, starting with when you would like to wake up for your best day and ending when you would like to go to sleep.

The second column is where you enter how you would prefer to best spend those half-hour time slots. If you need to, combine rows in the table. For example, if part of your best day is taking a walk from 8:30 to 9:30, merge the 8:30 and 9:00 rows. If it would work best for you, create one table for a best weekday and another for a best weekend day.

The next step is to fill in the realities of your cancer plan and other commitments. Perhaps just after your diagnosis and during your treatments, you couldn't go to work, but now you're back half time. Fill in the time slots needed to prepare for, travel to/from, and be at work. Or perhaps you're still going through chemotherapy infusions and need to be at the cancer center from 9:00 to 1:00 each day—fill that in. Or perhaps, you know that at least for now, you hit the energy wall mid-afternoon and find it difficult to get anything done. Be realistic and note the time slots that normally happens— fill that in with "nap" or "watch TV" or with whatever you judge to be the best use of that time.

The slots that remain open are the discretionary time you have to fill in your non-cancer plan. This is where the key elements come in. If you need to, go back in the chapter and review the elements. Figure out the key-element activities you want to include in your best-day time slots.

You may want to fill best-day time slots by pursuing a passion. How about an hour gardening? Or having friends over to play bridge (also positive for connectedness)?

You may want to spend time giving back. How about returning to volunteering at the local food pantry or leading a support group at which you used to be a participant at your cancer support center?

You may want to focus on intellectual growth. How about finally taking that evening class you've wanted to attend or spending an hour in the evening reading the latest book by your favorite author?

Key element activities can make your day and your life better. Isn't that the objective?

This approach enables you to be mindful about how you would spend your best day. It's written down, right in front of you. Now, compare your best day to how you're currently spending your days. The intent is to move from where you are to where you want to be. This transition doesn't need to be all at once, but it's important to get yourself moving in the right direction.

When you're pretty far along on your best day planning, take a look at your best week. Create another chart to include all seven days. The reason you want to do this is that there are some activities that may be part of a best day but not every day. An example may be exercising. For your wellbeing, you may include exercise in your best day plan, but you would likely not work out every day. Envisioning your best week would enable you to schedule your days and times of exercise and build them into your plans.

When you're ready, you can then move on to your best year plan. You may enjoy traveling for sightseeing or visiting out-of-town family. But that would not appropriately fit in your best day or best week plan. Create a simple table with column one being the months and column two being what you would want to do in the appropriate month. For example, we plan on visiting our son and his family, who live in Boston, a couple of times each year. Another example is an annual book festival that occurs here in St. Louis during the first couple of weeks in November. Attending its author programs is built into our best year plan.

You may never fully reach your best day/week/year plans, but always striving to do so is energizing and plays a role in building hope. You will also quickly note that circumstances change requiring that you update your plans. We'll look at the planning concept of "Renewal" later in the chapter.

Before we go on, one more reminder—in everyone's best interest, it will be helpful for both the survivor and loved ones to have their individual plans and have the crucial conversations to make sure that the plans overlap when they should.

Making Life Changes

"How wonderful it is that nobody need wait a single moment before starting to improve the world." Anne Frank wrote that. What changes would you not "wait a single moment" to make in your world?

This non-cancer life planning tool is another that makes good use of the key elements to help you decide what changes to make. It's time for another two-column table. In the first column, list the ten key elements, one per row. In the blanks in the second column, you'll be entering those things you wish to change in your life to be doing better in each key element.

One way to approach deciding what changes you'll make is to answer these two questions. "What things would I like to start in my life to improve my key elements?" "What things in my life would I stop that are getting in the way of improving my key elements?"

Fill out one or two start/stop items for each key element, then scan your list and pick two that you think will make the biggest difference to you and are doable. Work on making those changes before picking others to address. Most who try to take on too much at once find it difficult to do so. In regards to the difficulty many of us have in making changes, refer to "Skill, Will, and Support" in the "Planning" section before Chapter 8.

Here are some examples of start/stop changes for the key element they address:

> ➤ Growth: Stop watching more than an hour of television each day. Note: There is nothing fundamentally wrong with TV unless you are watching too much to the exclusion of more beneficial activities. The opportunity is to replace the passive TV time.

➢ Wellbeing: Start taking a daily walk.

➢ Attitude: Stop spending as much time with Susan, who is constantly complaining and whining about something.

➢ Planning: Start my bucket jars.

➢ Connectedness: Start attending the local cancer support group meetings.

➢ Passions: Start playing bridge at least twice per month.

One final thought on this tool—it should mesh well with the development of your best-day plan. For example, if you decide to start taking that daily walk, build it into your best day. If you choose to start playing bridge more often, build it into your best week.

Renewal

Even before you or a loved one was diagnosed, you experienced changing life circumstances, sometimes for the better and sometimes not. And you learned that whether you do so mindfully or not, when circumstances change, so does your life plan.

You meet the love of your life. A dear grandparent passes away. You get accepted into your preferred college. You get cut from your high school team. Your first grandchild is born. You get downsized during a corporate merger. Your investments rise or fall during a boom or bust. You are diagnosed with cancer. You are in remission. Life circumstances change.

Hopefully by now, you've embraced the idea that it is better to thoughtfully develop both your cancer and non-cancer plans—and to write them down. It's also better to mindfully renew those plans when circumstances warrant.

Renewal is more of a planning concept than a tool, and it applies to any of the planning methods you've chosen to use, even if you've created your own and even if you've chosen not to write them down.

There are several ideal times to review your current plan and renew it. Clearly, one of those times is when there is a significant change in circumstances, whether positive or negative. Another is when you are transitioning from one cancer stage to another, such as entering treatment or moving into post-treatment. Perhaps it's time for plan renewal if you find yourself having more than the normal difficulty coping with your emotions. And if nothing has changed, but it's been a while since you last modified your plan, invest some energy in deciding if and how to renew it.

Create a cancer plan? Absolutely. Create a non-cancer life plan? Absolutely. Review and renew them? Absolutely.

Resilience Muscles

The United States Army has a program called "Comprehensive Soldier Fitness" that addresses five aspects (physical, family, social, spiritual, emotional) of developing "Stronger Minds—Stronger Bodies."

One of the courses they provide is a 10-day program called "Master Resilience Training." The program defines resiliency as "the ability to grow and thrive in the face of challenges and bounce back from adversity." The premise of the course, which is based on studies at the University of Pennsylvania, is that an individual's resilience can be built. It's easy to understand how it would be important for military leaders to build resilience. It is equally easy to understand why that would also be important for cancer survivors and their loved ones.

Encouragingly, the concepts we've reviewed throughout the book to help us navigate cancer are consistent with the things taught in the Army program to build resilience:

> ➢ Acknowledge the reality of the setback.
> ➢ Sort out what you can and cannot control, then focus on what you can.
> ➢ Build deep relationships with those who can help you, then don't be afraid to ask for help, trusting your support team to do what's right for you.
> ➢ Embrace change—view a potentially traumatic circumstance as an opportunity to learn and plan around.
> ➢ Foster a hopeful attitude.
> ➢ Build and sustain the energy you'll need, which includes listening to your body about when it's time to rest, relax, and recharge.

These are easier said than done, and even when we do them, it may take a while to develop our resilience muscles. But that's what we've been doing together throughout the book. We have acknowledged the reality of our cancer, its treatment, and the emotions that ensue. We have recognized the importance of being hopeful and learned how to build hope. And we have done the planning, both our cancer plan and our non-cancer plan, thereby *Balancing Reality and Hope.*

Appendix

Cancer Statistics

In Chapter 1, we briefly referred to cancer statistics. This is a more detailed view of those data. Did you know?

➢ The percentage of the U.S. population who will be diagnosed is expected to increase—the projections are that greater than 50% of those born after 1960 will have cancer in their lifetime. The reasons for the increase include improvement in diagnostic capabilities and the aging of the population. Cancer is often age-related—the vast majority of those diagnosed are over 65 years old, and this segment of the population is expected to increase by about 50% by 2030.

➢ If you are reading this book because you are a newly diagnosed cancer survivor, you are among approximately 1.7 million new cases in the United States each year, a number also expected to rise.

➢ The number of new cancer cases globally each year is approximately 14 million, and this number is predicted to increase to nearly 24 million by 2030.

➢ Your survivorship makes you one of the nearly 14.5 million Americans with a history of cancer that are alive at any given time.

➢ There are about 600,000 deaths attributed to cancer in the U.S. each year and approximately 8.2 million worldwide.

➢ Nearly 170 million years of healthy life are lost to cancer globally each year.

➢ The effects of cancer are more than health related. There are also huge costs associated with the disease. We spend about $80 billion each year in the U.S. on direct medical costs (such as office visits, hospital outpatient tests and procedures, and inpatient hospital stays). These costs don't take into account cancer-related expenses at home, lost productivity in the workplace, or the cost of administering the cancer-related health care system.

Pretty bleak? Yes. Is the news all bad? Absolutely not. Did you know?

- ➤ The National Institutes of Health report that from 1975 to 2007:
    - ○ the mortality rate for all cancers dropped from 199 deaths per 100,000 population to 178 despite an increased incidence rate from 400 to 461 per 100,000
    - ○ the five-year relative survival rate for all cancers combined increased from 50% to approximately 68%--attributed to earlier diagnoses and enhancements in treatment
        > Note: "relative survival" is the percentage of people alive five years after a cancer diagnosis, divided by the percentage expected to be alive in the absence of cancer, based on normal life expectancy.
    - ○ the five-year relative survival rates for the most common cancers are up significantly: breast—90%, prostate—100%, colorectal—67%, bladder—81% (lung cancer, still among the most prevalent, retains only a 16% five-year relative survival rate)
- ➤ Since 2007, cancer mortality has continued to drop at the rate of 1.8% per year in men and 1.4% per year in women.

Children—Some More Data

Pediatric cancers are considered those in survivors under 15 years of age. Similar to cancer in general, there is the reality of the prevalence and effects of the disease and of the hope engendered by the progress that has been made. Did you know?

- ➤ Over 10,000 children will be diagnosed with cancer each year in the U.S.
- ➤ Approximately 1,250 children will die from cancer each year. Cancer is the #2 cause of death among children.
- ➤ The average age of a child diagnosed with cancer is six.
- ➤ There are nearly 410,000 people in the U.S. today who have survived a childhood cancer.

> ➤ The five-year relative survival rate for children diagnosed with all cancers was 58% in the mid-1970's and was up to 83% by 2011.
> ➤ The cancer mortality rate for children has dropped 1.6% per year since 2010.

ABOUT THE AUTHOR

Since retiring from the Procter & Gamble Company as a Director of Worldwide Quality Assurance, Alan Spector has authored six books prior to *Cancer: Balancing Reality and Hope*, founded three businesses, spoken around the country and blogged extensively about the non-financial aspects of retirement planning, and is a strategic planning consultant. He continues to play baseball with "kids his own age" in local leagues and in tournaments around the country and has played internationally. Spector is also a gym rat, nonprofit board member, community volunteer, avid crossword puzzle solver, and most importantly, the active and proud grandfather of four. He lives in St. Louis with his wife, Ann, with whom he travels extensively.

In 2010, Spector became part of the cancer community in two ways. He was diagnosed with Chronic Lymphocytic Leukemia, and he began to apply his strategic planning consultancy to major cancer institutions across the country.

Contact the author for special quantity discounts

Alan Spector

BBallNever2Old@aol.com

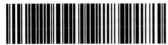

Made in the USA
Columbia, SC
19 April 2019